Empowering Your Journey:
Strategies and Stories for Transformative
Health and Wellness

BECOMING AN UNSTOPPABLE
WOMAN IN HEALTH & WELLNESS

PART
2

ADRIANA LUNA CARLOS AND HANNA OLIVAS

ALONG WITH 13 INSPIRING AUTHORS

ISBN: 978-1-964619-68-2

TABLE OF CONTENTS

INTRODUCTION

Welcome to **Becoming an Unstoppable Woman in Health & Wellness – Part 2: Empowering Your Journey - Strategies and Stories for Transformative Health & Wellness**, a powerful collection of stories, wisdom, and practical advice designed to inspire you on your own health journey. This anthology is a testament to the resilience, strength, and determination that women possess in the pursuit of better health and wellness.

Within these pages, you will meet remarkable women who have faced challenges, overcome obstacles, and emerged stronger, wiser, and more empowered. Each story offers a unique perspective, yet all are united by one common thread: the unwavering commitment to living a life of health, vitality, and fulfillment.

The women featured in this book share their most personal experiences, offering valuable insights and strategies that have helped them take control of their well-being. Their words will encourage you to make informed, intentional choices—whether it's cultivating a healthier mindset, adopting new fitness routines, embracing balanced nutrition, or prioritizing self-care.

As you read these powerful accounts, you will not only find inspiration but also practical tools you can apply to your own life. From overcoming adversity to embracing self-love, these stories will empower you to become the unstoppable woman you were always meant to be.

Let this book be your guide as you embark on your own health and wellness journey. May it remind you that resilience, courage, and a commitment to your well-being can transform your life in ways you never thought possible. The path to becoming an unstoppable woman is within your reach—take the first step today.

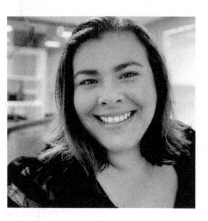

Adriana Luna Carlos

Founder and CEO of SHE RISES STUDIOS & FENIX TV

https://www.linkedin.com/in/adriana-luna-carlos/
https://www.facebook.com/adrianalunacarlos
https://www.instagram.com/sherisesstudios_llc/
https://www.sherisesstudios.com/
https://fenixtv.app/

Adriana Luna Carlos is an accomplished web and graphic designer, author, and mentor with a passion for helping women succeed in life and business. With over 10 years of experience in graphic and web arts, Adriana has built a reputation as an innovative leader and entrepreneur. In 2020, she co-founded She Rises Studios, a multi-digital media company and publishing house that has helped countless clients achieve their branding and marketing goals. In 2023, she co-created FENIX TV, an online streaming platform that showcases stories of people breaking barriers, shattering stereotypes, and triumphing against the odds.

As an advocate for women's success, Adriana challenges her clients and mentees to strive for nothing less than excellence. She has a deep understanding of the insecurities and challenges that women often face in the business world and provides the guidance and resources needed to overcome them. Her success as a business leader and entrepreneur has made her a sought-after mentor and speaker at events around the world.

Through her work, Adriana has demonstrated a commitment to creating opportunities for women to succeed in business and life. Her passion for innovation, leadership, and women's empowerment has made her a respected figure in the business community, and her impact will undoubtedly continue to inspire and empower women for years to come.

Embracing Health with Heart

By Adriana Luna Carlos

When I think about what it means to be unstoppable in health and wellness, it's less about having perfect habits and more about showing up for myself every day—mind, body, and soul. This journey is a commitment to my well-being, even on the days when I don't feel like it. And believe me, there are days like that. Over time, I've come to see that being unstoppable isn't about having it all figured out. It's about staying open, embracing the ups and downs, and learning to really value myself along the way.

My journey hasn't been without significant health struggles, both physical and mental. These battles are deeply personal, and this is the first time I'm speaking about some of them publicly. I've faced long, heavy periods—at one point, they lasted for an entire year without a break, accompanied by blood clots. This condition has impacted me physically in obvious ways, causing fatigue, anemia, and other health challenges that make everyday life harder. Eventually, this led to struggles with infertility, which has been one of the most heartbreaking parts of my journey. Having children has always been a dream of mine, and grappling with the possibility that it may not happen has taken a toll on my mental health. I've faced depression, feeling at times like my body has betrayed me and questioning my future. But I've come to understand that resilience isn't about having a perfect life. It's about picking yourself up and finding strength in yourself, even on the hardest days.

About a year ago, I was also diagnosed with Type 2 Diabetes, a condition that introduced new challenges into my life. With diabetes came a complication called Diabetic Gastroparesis, which causes unpredictable and painful digestive issues. It's been a frightening experience; there have been times when I've nearly collapsed, struggling to get my body stable during flare-ups. I've had to rush to the hospital more than four times, feeling close to death and powerless to stop what was happening. These moments have not only taken a toll on my body but have also been exhausting mentally. Facing down this invisible illness over and over again tests my resilience and reminds me daily of the strength it takes to keep going.

Redefining Wellness for Myself

Starting out, I approached wellness the way I approached most things in life—goal by goal. Maybe I wanted to feel healthier or have more energy. But as I went deeper, I realized it was about something much more profound. Wellness wasn't just about what I did; it was about how I felt. I wasn't chasing perfection; I was chasing the feeling of being grounded and at peace.

The real shift came when I stopped focusing so much on results and started caring more about how I felt inside. I realized wellness was not about squeezing into a particular mold. Instead, it was about honoring my unique self, treating my body kindly, and recognizing my own worth. This shift made all the difference, allowing me to enjoy the process instead of constantly striving for some "ideal."

Being unstoppable in health and wellness has meant building resilience. It's about learning how to bounce back on the tough days, the tired days, the "I just don't want to" days. It's about showing up consistently, even if I don't feel like going all out. I found out that the real magic comes from small, steady actions over time.

For a while, I thought resilience was about pushing myself harder. But now I see it's about being kind to myself, too. When setbacks happen (and they always do), I remind myself that each day is a new chance. I've learned that resilience means picking myself up, dusting myself off, and knowing that it's okay to take things slow as long as I keep moving forward.

Embracing Self-Care and Finding Joy in It

For me, self-care isn't a luxury; it's a necessity. Once I stopped feeling guilty about taking time for myself, I started to thrive. I used to think self-care was indulgent, but now I see it as essential to being my best self. Taking care of myself helps me stay grounded and gives me the energy I need to be there for others.

Self-care also taught me to slow down and be mindful. I started meditating, journaling, and just taking a moment to breathe every now and then. I've come to see these quiet moments as gifts—opportunities to reconnect with myself and remind myself why I'm on this journey. It's in these moments that I find my balance again.

One of the biggest shifts in my wellness journey has been learning to nourish my body from a place of love, not restriction. I used to view food as something to control, but now I see it as fuel, a way of honoring my body. Choosing foods that make me feel energized, strong, and healthy became a natural part of caring for myself.

And then there's movement. I stopped looking at exercise as something I "had to do" and started doing things I genuinely enjoyed. I experimented with different kinds of movement until I found what felt good for me—whether it's yoga, hiking, or dancing. I learned that wellness doesn't have to be a chore. In fact, it's even better when it's fun.

Taking Care of My Mind and Emotions, Too

Physical wellness is great, but I also had to take care of my mind and heart. Becoming unstoppable meant confronting limiting beliefs, embracing self-compassion, and letting go of old patterns. This meant training myself to stop the negative self-talk and replace it with a little kindness. I started talking to myself the way I'd talk to a friend, and wow—what a difference that made.

Emotionally, it's been about letting myself feel without judgment. I've learned to lean into my emotions rather than pushing them aside, and I've reached out for support when I need it. Allowing myself to be vulnerable has been one of the most empowering parts of this journey. It's a reminder that true strength isn't about holding everything together; it's about being real and honest with myself.

As I've embraced health and wellness for myself, I've found so much joy in sharing it with others. I want every woman to know that wellness is for her, too—that she's worth the time, the effort, and the love. Supporting other women on their journeys has reminded me that we're stronger together. When we lift each other up, there's no limit to what we can achieve.

Wellness doesn't have to be a solo journey. By connecting with others, we build a community of support, inspiration, and shared growth. I've learned so much from other women who have been on this path, and it's shown me that wellness is as much about community as it is about self.

The Journey is the Destination

Being unstoppable in health and wellness isn't about hitting a certain goal; it's about choosing, day after day, to care for myself in meaningful ways. This journey has shown me that I am resilient, capable, and worthy of living a life of health and happiness. I know I'll never "arrive" at some final point in my wellness journey, and that's okay. Every day, every small step, is part of the journey, and that's what makes it so rewarding.

So, to every woman out there reading this, remember: you're worth the commitment. Start small if you need to. Find the things that bring you joy and keep you grounded. Embrace the journey as it comes, and know that each step forward, no matter how tiny, is a victory in itself.

This journey of wellness and health isn't just about what we do. It's about who we're becoming along the way—stronger, kinder, and more connected to ourselves. You are unstoppable, and you're worthy of every ounce of health and happiness this world has to offer. Go after it, and make your wellness journey your own.

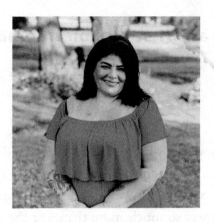

Hanna Olivas

Founder and CEO of SHE RISES STUDIOS

https://www.linkedin.com/company/she-rises-studios/
https://www.facebook.com/sherisesstudios
https://www.instagram.com/sherisesstudios_llc/
www.SheRisesStudios.com

Author, Speaker, and Founder. Hanna was born and raised in Las Vegas, Nevada, and has paved her way to becoming one of the most influential women of 2022. Hanna is the co-founder of She Rises Studios and the founder of the Brave & Beautiful Blood Cancer Foundation. Her journey started in 2017 when she was first diagnosed with Multiple Myeloma, an incurable blood cancer. Now more than ever, her focus is to empower other women to become leaders because The Future is Female. She is currently traveling and speaking publicly to women to educate them on entrepreneurship, leadership, and owning the female power within.

Becoming an Unstoppable Woman Through Health and Wellness

By Hanna Olivas

Health and wellness have often been misunderstood as merely physical aspects of our lives. We are conditioned to think about exercise routines, diets, and losing weight. However, the true essence of health and wellness encompasses so much more than just the physical body. It's about the alignment of your mind, body, soul, and spirit, a journey that leads to the discovery of your truest self. This chapter is not just about how to maintain health and wellness—it's about becoming an unstoppable woman in your own life by fully embracing the connection between your mental, emotional, physical, and spiritual well-being.

As I've walked my own path toward health and wellness, I've come to realize one profound truth: Health and wellness are not destinations; they are lifelong journeys. It's not about perfection, but rather, about progress. It's about being kind to ourselves, showing up every day with love, and embracing each moment with the intention of nurturing all parts of our being. And more than anything, it's about listening to our inner voice, the one that tells us what we truly need to thrive.

"To become unstoppable, you must first honor the place where you are right now and trust that every step you take toward your health and wellness is part of your divine journey."

The Mind: Nourishing Mental Health

When we speak of health, the mind is often the most neglected part. Yet, mental health is the foundation of our entire well-being. If our mind is not healthy—if it is cluttered with self-doubt, stress, and negative thoughts—it becomes nearly impossible to take care of the other aspects of our health.

Becoming an unstoppable woman requires nurturing your mental health by silencing the inner critic that tells you you're not enough or that you're failing. It's about recognizing the power of your thoughts and how they shape your reality. Your mind is the garden of your life, and what you plant there—be it love, positivity, or self-belief—will bloom into the life you live.

Taking care of your mental health means giving yourself the grace to slow down when you need to. It means creating boundaries that protect your energy and spending time doing things that bring you peace and joy. Meditation, journaling, and mindfulness practices are all tools that help quiet the chaos in our minds and connect us to the present moment, where real change begins.

"The most profound transformation begins when we recognize that our thoughts are not just passive reflections of our experiences—they are the architects of our future."

Mental wellness also involves self-awareness—being mindful of what drains you, what fills you with anxiety, and what brings you joy. When you start paying attention to the thoughts that cycle through your mind, you begin to see how they impact your emotional and physical health. Learning to let go of negative thinking patterns and replace them with positive, affirming thoughts is essential to becoming an unstoppable woman.

The Body: Honoring the Physical Vessel

Our body is the vehicle through which we experience life. It is the vessel that carries our spirit, our dreams, and our purpose. To become an unstoppable woman, we must honor our body as a sacred temple—one that deserves to be nourished, cared for, and respected.

There's an inherent wisdom in the body that we often overlook. Our body speaks to us in subtle ways—through fatigue, tension, and even illness—telling us what it needs. The journey to health and wellness begins with listening to your body's cues and giving it what it asks for, whether that's more rest, movement, or nourishment.

Exercise and movement are not just about weight loss or looking a certain way. They are about building strength, endurance, and resilience. They are about connecting with your body in a way that empowers you and makes you feel alive. When you move your body with love—whether it's through yoga, walking, dancing, or lifting weights—you're not just working on your physical health, you're strengthening the bond between your mind, body, and soul.

But just as important as movement is rest. We live in a culture that glorifies hustle, pushing our bodies to the brink of exhaustion. But true wellness requires balance—knowing when to push and when to rest. Rest is not a weakness; it is a vital part of health. Sleep is when our body repairs itself, when our mind processes and releases stress, and when our soul reconnects with the quiet peace it needs.

"To be unstoppable, you must honor your body by recognizing that rest is not a luxury; it is essential for your growth and well-being."

Nourishment is another key aspect of physical health. What we feed our bodies directly impacts how we feel mentally and emotionally. A balanced, whole-food diet is more than just fuel—it's a form of self-love. Choosing foods that nourish your body, mind, and soul helps create harmony within and promotes long-term health.

Becoming unstoppable means tuning into your body's needs and fueling it with intention and care. It means rejecting the societal pressure to look a certain way and instead embracing the beauty, strength, and power that your body holds, exactly as it is right now.

The Soul: Connecting with Your Inner Essence

Wellness for the soul is about connecting with the deepest parts of yourself. It's about nourishing the part of you that is timeless, the part that holds your dreams, passions, and sense of purpose. Becoming an unstoppable woman means tuning into your soul's voice and living a life that is aligned with who you truly are.

Too often, we disconnect from our souls, becoming lost in the noise of the world, the expectations of others, and the hustle of daily life. But true wellness requires time to quiet the outside world and listen to the whispers of your soul. It's in these quiet moments that we reconnect with our deepest desires and understand the path we are meant to walk.

Self-reflection, prayer, meditation, and creative expression are all ways to nurture your soul. These practices allow you to connect with your inner essence, to explore who you are beyond the labels and roles that you play in life. When you nurture your soul, you step into your truest self—the unstoppable woman who is guided by her heart and aligned with her purpose.

"The soul knows the way. When you connect with your inner essence, you find the strength and wisdom to navigate every challenge and rise above every obstacle."

Nurturing your soul also means giving yourself permission to follow your passions. So many women set aside their own dreams to care for others or meet the expectations of society. But to be truly unstoppable, you must honor the things that light you up inside. Pursue the things that make your soul come alive, whether it's painting, writing, traveling, or helping others. When you live in alignment with your passions, you become unstoppable because you are living a life that is true to who you are.

The Spirit: Embracing a Higher Purpose

Well-being is incomplete without spiritual health. While we each have our own understanding of spirituality, it's the connection with something greater than ourselves that brings peace and fulfillment. Whether you call it God, the universe, or a higher power, this connection is what grounds us, gives us perspective, and reminds us that we are part of something much larger than ourselves.

Spiritual wellness is about trusting in the journey, even when it's difficult. It's about recognizing that every challenge you face is an opportunity for growth and transformation. When you are connected to your spiritual self, you understand that you are never truly alone. There is a divine energy guiding you, supporting you, and helping you become the unstoppable woman you are meant to be.

"To be unstoppable, you must trust the journey, knowing that every step you take is leading you toward the woman you are destined to become."

Spiritual health also involves living with intention and purpose. It's about asking yourself, "What is my purpose? How can I contribute to the world?" When you live with a sense of purpose, every action you take, no matter how small, becomes meaningful. You wake up each day with the knowledge that you are living in alignment with your higher purpose, and this gives you the strength to persevere through any challenge.

Living with spiritual health also means cultivating gratitude. Gratitude shifts our focus from what we lack to what we have. It reminds us of the abundance that exists in our lives and connects us to the beauty of the present moment. Gratitude is a powerful force for transformation, and when practiced regularly, it creates a sense of peace and fulfillment.

Becoming Unstoppable: The Journey of Self-Love

At the heart of health and wellness is self-love. To become an unstoppable woman, you must love yourself fiercely, unapologetically, and without condition. Self-love is the foundation upon which all other aspects of well-being are built. Without it, we cannot truly care for our mind, body, soul, or spirit.

Self-love means recognizing your worth and knowing that you are enough exactly as you are. It means honoring your body, nurturing your mind, and connecting with your soul because you know you deserve to be cared for. Self-love is not selfish; it is the most profound act of kindness you can give yourself.

"Becoming unstoppable begins with loving yourself fully—embracing every part of who you are and treating yourself with the kindness and compassion you so freely give to others."

To practice self-love, you must set boundaries that protect your energy, say no when you need to, and prioritize your own well-being without guilt. It is to forgive yourself for past mistakes, to release the need for perfection, and to celebrate the progress you make along the way.

Self-love is also about trusting yourself. It's about knowing that you are capable, strong, and resilient. Trusting yourself means believing in your ability to overcome obstacles, rise above challenges, and create the life you desire. When you trust yourself, you become unstoppable.

The Power of Self-Care: Nurturing Yourself Daily

Becoming an unstoppable woman in health and wellness also means embracing self-care, not as an indulgence but as a necessary part of your life. Self-care is how we recharge, how we fill ourselves back up so that we can give to others and to the world.

Self-care comes in many forms: rest, relaxation, creative outlets, laughter, and simply doing the things that make your heart happy. It's about making yourself a priority in your own life. When you practice self-care, you're telling yourself that you matter and that your well-being is worth investing in.

Self-care can be as simple as a warm bath, a cup of tea in silence, or a few minutes spent breathing deeply in meditation. It can also be a more structured routine—like regular exercise, nourishing meals, or setting aside time for spiritual practices. Whatever form it takes, self-care is the foundation of your health and wellness journey, and it allows you to be the unstoppable force you were meant to be.

"To be unstoppable, you must take the time to nurture yourself, to care for your own needs, and to fill your own cup so that you can give from a place of abundance."

Wellness as a Way of Life

Health and wellness are not destinations, but ways of life. They are the practices, habits, and choices that we make each day that allow us to live fully and joyfully. They are about being in harmony with yourself—mentally, emotionally, physically, and spiritually.

The journey to becoming an unstoppable woman in your health and wellness is about making a commitment to yourself. It's about showing up for yourself every day, even when it's hard, or even when life gets busy. It's about believing that you deserve to live a life of vitality, joy, and purpose.

Becoming unstoppable means embracing the process, trusting the journey, and knowing that every step you take toward better health and wellness is a step toward becoming the best version of yourself.

Conclusion: Your Health and Wellness Are the Keys to Your Power

As women, we often give so much of ourselves to others that we forget to nurture our own well-being. But the truth is, we cannot be unstoppable in our lives—whether in our careers, relationships, or personal endeavors—if we are not first unstoppable in our health and wellness.

Taking care of your mind, body, soul, and spirit is not just an act of self-preservation; it is an act of empowerment. When you prioritize your health and wellness, you become stronger, more resilient, and more capable of facing whatever life throws your way.

"Health and wellness are the keys to unlocking your true power. When you honor yourself—mind, body, soul, and spirit—you step into your full potential and become the unstoppable woman you were always meant to be."

Remember, this journey is not about perfection. It's about progress, self-love, and showing up for yourself every day. It's about embracing the ups and downs, trusting the process, and knowing that you are worthy of living a life of balance, health, and joy.

Becoming an unstoppable woman is not just about reaching a goal or hitting a milestone—it's about embodying a way of being that honors who you are in every moment of your life. And that journey begins with your health and wellness.

You have everything within you to become unstoppable, to live a life that is aligned with your highest self, and to thrive in every aspect of your being. All it takes is a commitment to love yourself, care for yourself, and nurture your mind, body, soul, and spirit.

Now, it's time to rise into the unstoppable woman that you are and to embrace the fullness of your health and wellness journey. You've got this!

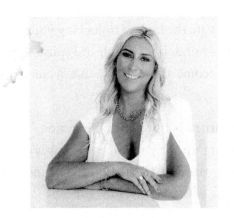

Marissa Warren

Hypnotherapist & Transformational Consultant

https://www.linkedin.com/in/marissawarren-hypnotherapist-transformationalconsultant/
https://www.facebook.com/marissa.warren.transformational
https://www.instagram.com/marissawarren_/
https://www.marissawarren.com/

Marissa is a hypnotherapist and transformational consultant working with RTT – Rapid Transformational Therapy, QHHT – Quantum Healing Hypnosis Technique, Somatic and Tantric embodiment, breathwork and sound healing and is also an international speaker and author.

Known as the clarity queen, Marissa has a phenomenal ability to tap deeply into people's subconscious to help them break free from internal limitations, negative patterns and behaviours and allow them to move into living their dream life and souls purpose.

Leaving you feeling empowered, living from infinite inner power and potential and stepping into the life and level of success you desire. Marissa will help you tap into your inner magic and utilise your inner resources to step up and shine.

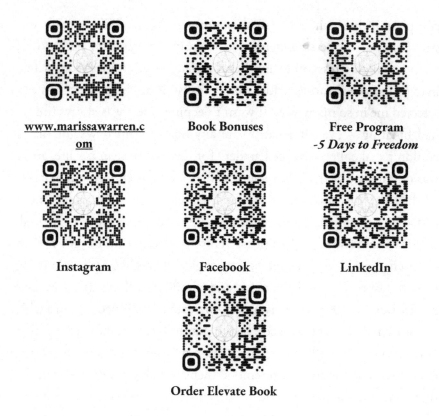

www.marissawarren.com

Book Bonuses

Free Program
-5 Days to Freedom

Instagram

Facebook

LinkedIn

Order Elevate Book

Bounce Back from Burnout: Recovery and Prevention Strategies to Help You Live Your Best Life

By Marissa Warren

If you have ever suffered from burnout, you'll know first-hand how hard and slow this can be to recover from and that this is something that you will need to regularly monitor to avoid reoccurring. I didn't even think burnout was a real thing until I suffered from it eight years ago.

I had ended a highly toxic relationship and was self-employed with three businesses – all in the start-up phase. One of those businesses was a complete money pit, and I had a mortgage to pay. To say life was stressful is an understatement! Throughout my career, I had moved from one high-stress job to another for many years and was completely living in survival mode; I just didn't realise it at the time. Stress has affected me in so many ways. I wasn't sleeping, and I was always tired. I had bloating – even if I hardly ate anything, I gained weight that I couldn't shake. I experienced anxiety for the first time in my life, and I was definitely not the best version of myself. I was cranky and irritable all the time, the opposite of the carefree, relaxed version I aim to be. I ended up a complete shell of myself – numbed out on all levels – mental, physical, emotional, and spiritual. This was truly a death and rebirth experience, and it felt like moving through this was like a phoenix rising from the ashes. I had to learn to feel and rebuild myself. It was like me and my life was a 1000-piece jigsaw puzzle that had been tipped out on a table and scattered all over the place. I had to put the pieces of me back together again, but they would never quite fit the same again. This was when I first discovered somatic and tantric embodiment and these modalities were the only thing that helped me to feel again and heal. This was a turning point in my life and one that would permanently impact the course of my life. It was because of this experience that I learnt the power of somatic embodiment work, how stress really affects the body, and why it is so important to live life in alignment with me and my sovereignty.

In today's fast-paced world and demanding daily life, burnout has become a common challenge for many people. Whether you have focused on your career, are a student, a parent, or all of the above, the constant demands of daily life can take a toll on your mental, physical, and emotional well-being. Burnout is not just about being tired; it's an overwhelming state of exhaustion and depletion that impacts all areas of your life. Burnout affects your ability to function, thrive, and enjoy life and keeps you stuck in survival mode, struggling to simply exist and make it through each day. When your in burnout it can feel like it will never end, however recovery from burnout is possible!

Burnout is a state of chronic physical and emotional exhaustion caused by prolonged periods of stress, which can be from work or life events.

Burnout slowly builds and develops over time, starting subtly and growing worse if not corrected. It involves feelings of exhaustion, detachment, a reduced sense of accomplishment, a lack of life purpose, feeling like you are just drifting and existing in life, with no motivation, high procrastination levels, and an inability to find joy in daily life or be fully present. For those experiencing burnout, you may feel emotionally drained, mentally fatigued, or even physically ill.

Recognising burnout can be challenging as the symptoms can appear as general stress or tiredness. Burnout does have common signs and characteristics that differ from normal fatigue.

Here are the signs to look out for:

Chronic Exhaustion

- Constantly waking up tired and struggling to get out of bed.
- Feeling physically and emotionally drained, even after a good night's sleep.
- Inability to fall asleep.
- The feeling of exhaustion is persistent, affecting your energy levels throughout the day.

Detachment and Cynicism

- Hypercritical of self and others.
- Start distancing yourself emotionally from work, family, or social activities.
- An increasing sense of cynicism towards your responsibilities.
- You feel detached from people and life.

Reduced Performance and Accomplishment

- Tasks that once felt manageable now seem overwhelming.
- A drop in productivity.
- Feeling ineffective or incompetent.
- You feel that the harder you work, the less results you are achieving.

Mental and Physical Fatigue

- Mental clarity becomes clouded, making decision-making and concentration difficult.
- Experiencing physical symptoms like headaches, muscle tension, or digestive problems.
- Constantly feeling tired and fatigued.
- Lacking motivation.
- Procrastination increases.

Emotional Overwhelm

- Feelings of anxiety, irritability, or hopelessness increase.
- Feeling emotionally fragile and on the verge of breaking down.
- Heightened emotions.
- Easily triggered by others.

Sleep Disturbances

- Insomnia or restless sleep patterns.
- Despite long hours in bed, you may wake up feeling unrested.
- Constantly tired, but unable to sleep well.
- Frequent waking through the night.
- Energy slumps in the afternoon.
- Sluggish to wake up.
- Scrolling on your phone or binging on TV until late at night.

Loss of Passion or Purpose

- Activities that once brought you joy or meaning now feel unfulfilling.
- Feeling disconnected from your sense of purpose.
- Questioning your daily existence.
- Uncertain about the future.
- Unable to set goals – both short and long-term.

Burnout affects not only your work and productivity; it ripples through into all aspects of your life, from your relationships to your physical and emotional health. The longer burnout goes unchecked and unmanaged, the more detrimental it becomes to your quality of life.

Burnout creates and is a by-product of high levels of stress in the body, triggering the fight, flight, or freeze response with in the body. This can create a myriad of issues which can include:

Mental Health

Burnout can increase mental health conditions like anxiety and depression. The chronic stress burnout generates can lead to feelings of hopelessness, lack of motivation, low self-esteem, decreased self-confidence, and a questioning of life's purpose. When your mental health suffers, it becomes harder to see a way out of burnout, creating a cycle that is difficult to break. You end up stuck in looping thoughts, stuck in the pit of despair, repeating negative behaviours and actions without seeing a way out.

Physical Health

Prolonged exposure to stress impacts your body in so many significant ways. Stress hormones like cortisol and adrenaline are elevated during burnout, which can lead to high blood pressure, weight gain, and an increased risk of heart disease. It is also common to experience muscle tension, chronic pain, and digestive issues. You may also struggle with your diet as you are more likely to opt for quick and convenience foods, rather than meal-prep healthy and nutritious foods. The cravings for sugar and sweets can also increase, and with the affected sleep, you are more likely to gravitate towards late-night snacks or multiple cups of coffee throughout the day to give yourself an energy boost. While it may feel hard and almost insurmountable, you know that eating well will give you more energy, and even some gentle movements will help bring back energy and clear stagnation in the body.

Relationships

Burnout can make you irritable, withdrawn, and emotionally unavailable to the people around you. This can strain relationships with family, friends, and colleagues. With the increased exhaustion levels, it can feel like a struggle to socialise or engage with others, which only further isolates you from supportive networks that could help you recover. Making the time to connect, even if for a quick catch-up, can make you feel so much better. Human connection is crucial for getting you out of your head, breaking the looping thoughts, and moving you out of the inner world of purgatory that you feel stuck in.

Work and Productivity

At work, burnout manifests as decreased productivity, lack of creativity, and disengagement. This can create missed deadlines, reduced work quality, feelings of inadequacy, high levels of self-doubt and self-criticism, and even more stress. Burnout may also contribute to increased absenteeism due to taking time from stress-related illnesses or impaired presenteeism, where you're physically present but mentally checked out.

Emotional Well-Being

Emotionally, burnout can leave you feeling drained and numb. It is common to experience feelings of apathy, irritability, frustration, anger, and resentment, or it can also be common to struggle to feel any emotions at all. The inability to feel emotions or bodily sensations and the numbing out effect is a stress response in the body and is a result of the nervous system being impacted over a period of time, without the ability to reset during stressful times. Over time, burnout can erode your sense of self-worth and leave you feeling disconnected from your own emotions. Self-worth and self-belief are important resources to utilise. These help you to have the confidence to navigate life with increased resilience and also prioritise yourself.

Recovering from burnout requires intentional time and effort. While you may be tempted to push through the fatigue or feel the societal pressure to just keep going and suck it up or feel conditioned by the hustle culture, it's essential to prioritise your mental, emotional, and physical well-being and take steps to heal. What you don't feel, you can't heal.

Here are key strategies to help you bounce back from burnout:

Acknowledge the Problem

The first step to recovery is recognising that you are suffering from burnout. Denial or ignoring the issue will prolong your recovery and make the situation worse. Be honest with yourself about how you're feeling and accept that you need a break.

Seek Professional Support

Burnout can be overwhelming, and sometimes you need outside help to navigate it. Speaking with a professional who can provide you with tools to manage stress and cope with burnout. You don't need to suffer alone, and asking for help isn't a sign of weakness; it is a sign of strength. Having a support network in place can help you move out of burnout faster and prevent this from happening again.

Rest and Rejuvenate

Rest is essential to recover from burnout. This doesn't just mean physical rest but also mental and emotional relaxation. Take time off from work, if possible and invest time in activities and hobbies that bring you joy. Life doesn't need to be hard, and you can bring fun into even the mundane daily tasks. You've heard the saying on every flight, "Put your own mask on first". Taking time to prioritise self-care isn't selfish, it is selfless. When you take the time to fill your own self-love cup, you have more to overflow out to others. If you deplete yourself by being a people pleaser or always giving to others, you have nothing left to nourish yourself with.

Set Boundaries

Boundaries are critical in avoiding further stress. Learn to say no to additional responsibilities that can create more overwhelm for you. Clearly communicate with colleagues, friends, and family about your needs and limitations and ask for help. You don't need to suffer alone. When you have clear boundaries, it is easier to maintain standards for what is manageable for you and prevent burnout from reoccurring.

Reconnect with Your Purpose

Burnout can leave you feeling disconnected from your sense of purpose or have you questioning the meaning of your life. Take time to reflect on what truly matters to you. Feed your soul's nourishment through activities that align with your values, bring you joy and happiness, and reignite your passion in life by focusing on meaningful goals.

Practice Mindfulness and Relaxation Techniques

Mindfulness practices, like meditation, deep breathing exercises, and yoga, can help reduce stress and increase relaxation. Mindfulness helps you stay present in the moment, reducing anxiety and emotional overwhelm. It also brings your focus and attention back to what is true in the current moment, not the fabricated scenario in your mind.

Physical Activity and Movement

Physical activity is a powerful antidote to burnout. Exercise helps reduce stress hormones, boosts your mood, and improves energy levels. Even gentle activities like yoga, stretching, or walking can significantly enhance your recovery process. When you are feeling the full effects of burnout, it can feel incredibly hard to gather the energy to exercise, so start off small and build the intensity and frequency over time.

Improve Sleep Hygiene

Sleep is crucial for mental and physical recovery. Creating a consistent bedtime routine, avoiding stimulants like caffeine before bed, and creating a sleep-friendly environment by limiting screen time and reducing noise can provide amazing benefits for improving sleep quality. One of the worst things you can do is scroll on your phone until right up before you go to bed. This can affect the ability of your mind to be able to slip into the relaxation brain waves, delaying deep and restorative sleep.

Nourish Your Body

Nutrition plays an essential role in recovering from burnout and is a super boost to more energy, mental clarity, and motivation. Eating a healthy and balanced diet that eliminates processed foods can help restore your energy levels and improve your mood. If you eat a diet high in processed foods, your body has to work harder to digest these foods, draining even more of your already limited energy. Light and high-vibe foods like fruit and vegetables give you light and high-vibe energy in return.

Preventing burnout requires adopting sustainable habits and practices that protect your mental, physical, and emotional well-being. Prevention isn't about avoiding stress altogether but learning to utilise tools and resources to effectively manage this.

Here are ways to prevent burnout:

Prioritise Self-Care

By incorporating self-care practices into your daily life, you are giving yourself the gift of self-care and self-prioritisation. This could include exercise, reading, journaling, meditating, grounding in nature or spending time with loved ones. Taking care of yourself should be non-negotiable and part of your daily rituals and habits.

Set Realistic Expectations

Setting achievable goals and managing expectations is key to preventing burnout. If you are setting goals and pressure for yourself, give yourself the grace to adjust these as needed. Avoid overcommitting to tasks or responsibilities that stretch you too thin. Ask for help and delegate to spread the workload between others. While you may have a high capacity to take on and do a lot of work, you don't always need to. You don't need to do everything!

Build a Support System

Surround yourself with people who support and encourage you. Having a strong support network of friends, family, or colleagues can provide emotional support, guidance, and a sense of belonging. As humans, we thrive on social connections and real-life interactions. In a society that has created social media, now, more than ever, people are feeling isolated, disconnected and craving connection and closeness. Isolation can grow feelings of internal despair and keep you locked in your own inner world of misery or feeling you have no support and help and have to do everything on your own, which fuels the burnout feelings for longer.

Create Work-Life Balance

Striking and maintaining a balance between work and personal life is crucial. Make time for activities outside of work that nourish your soul, like hobbies, travel, or relaxation. Establish clear boundaries between your work and personal time to avoid overextending yourself and learn to say no, guilt-free. We tend to put so much pressure on ourselves to get everything done, but the to-do list never ends! In most cases, the workload and pressure we have created for ourselves are self-imposed and can be adjusted and lightened to make life easier for ourselves.

Learn Stress Management Techniques

Managing stress effectively is vital for healing from and preventing burnout. When you incorporate stress-reduction techniques, such as mindfulness, journaling, breathwork, exercise, or spending time in nature, into your daily life, it becomes much easier to live a life burnout-free. Feel all the feels! When we feel emotions that are intense, but shut these down, it can prevent you from moving through the stress response cycle and keeps trauma stored in the body. If you allow yourself to feel the range of emotions, you are allowing your body to follow its natural completion process, and you can regulate in a real-time response.

Stay Connected to Your Values

Invest time into activities that align with your personal values and passions. Doing work that is meaningful and fulfilling helps you to maintain motivation and reduces the risk of burnout. The more passionate you are about things, the more likely you are to want to do these and feel a sense of reward from them. When you live in true alignment with what makes your soul happy and how you want to be living, not how you've been societally conditioned to live life, you are free to create the life you desire to be living.

How to Create Daily Routines to Avoid Burnout and Live Your Best Life

Creating daily routines that prioritise your mental, emotional, physical, and spiritual well-being is one of the most effective ways to prevent burnout and live a happier, stress-free life. Daily routines provide a solid framework for nourishing yourself and staying on track with self-maintenance.

To avoid burnout and live your best life, try these tips:

- Start your day with intention. Begin with a mindfulness practice, like meditation or breathwork. This is great to centre into yourself and the present moment.
- Move your body. Exercise will move and increase the energy in your body.
- Create a gratitude practice and reflect on everything you are grateful for and set a positive tone for the day ahead.
- Establish time management standards. Try to batch your tasks and leave time in your day for downtime.
- Rest and pause throughout the day. Recharging helps you stay focused throughout the day and avoid energy depletion.
- Set boundaries for work/life balance.
- Enjoy a digital detox and spend time away from social media, devices, and screens, especially at least one hour before bedtime. This will help to give you a good night's sleep.
- Journaling helps to get the thoughts out of your head and gives you a new sense of clarity.

- Prioritise relaxation practices and make this a part of your daily routine. This will help keep your nervous system calm and prevent burnout from reoccurring.
- Give yourself a weekly check-in to assess how your stress levels are and if you are feeling any burnout. Adjust as needed and make adaptations to keep you feeling calm and in control of your daily life.
- Create space in your daily life for fun.
- Nourishing nutrition through healthy balanced meals to fuel your body and mind.

It is possible to live your best life after burnout, and you can recover from this. Burnout is a serious condition, but this isn't permanent. By understanding the signs and symptoms and acknowledging the impact on your life, you can take proactive steps towards recovery. You can bounce back from burnout and rebuild a life full of purpose, balance, joy, and passion. Prevention is key, along with integrating self-care, mindfulness, and daily routines, you can easily protect yourself from burnout. You are worthy and deserving of living your best life and a life where your mental, physical, and emotional harmony and equilibrium are a priority. The recovery from burnout isn't just about healing; it's about reclaiming your life and living it to the fullest every single day.

Meet Marissa, known as the "Clarity Queen". Marissa is a globally renowned clinical hypnotherapist and transformational consultant working with RTT – Rapid Transformational Therapy, QHHT – Quantum Healing Hypnosis Technique, PTSD Hypnotherapy, Somatic and Tantric embodiment, breathwork, and sound healing. Marissa is also an international speaker and author.

Marissa truly embodies these modalities in her daily life and has used these herself to heal from trauma, make major life changes, create lasting transformations, and align with her soul's purpose. This work is truly the work she is here to do, and it is her life's purpose. Marissa now uses these modalities with her clients to help them break free from past limitations to live their best lives.

Marissa aims to leave her clients feeling empowered, living from their infinite inner power and potential and stepping into the life and level of success they truly desire. Everything you need is already within you, and Marissa will help you tap into this inner magic and utilise your inner resources to step up and shine.

Rapid Transformational therapy is a fantastic modality combining hypnosis, cognitive behavioural therapy, NLP – neurolinguistic programming and psychotherapy together to really get to the root cause of whatever is going on and creating an issue or limitation in life, then release this and then recode and rewire the subconscious to operate in a more aligned and conducive way to help move the client into living the life they have always wanted to live and to create the life they truly desire. It's super effective for achieving amazing results. I often find clients that come to me after trying it all: they've seen everyone and spent countless hours in therapy and counselling and are at their last resort. The thing I love the most about this work is the changes that occur and ripple out into many areas of life. This is a super effective treatment and whereas normal hypnotherapy may require 4 – 6 or more sessions for an issue or area of concern, the method of RTT can achieve deeper results in 1 – 3 sessions. This is due to the therapy modalities used during hypnosis.

QHHT is working with past life regression. There is so much that can be carried through, which can all impact health and harmony in this current and daily life. Accessing deeper parts of yourself helps to gain a deeper understanding into yourself and allows you to tap into the inner wisdom of YOU! This can be a great modality to release past karma or burdens and go on a deeper inner journey of self-exploration. This is a phenomenal option for those seeking their life purpose – knowing that there is a deep feeling of wanting more from life and knowing that you are destined for more in this life.

PTSD Hypnotherapy uses clinical hypnotherapy to help eliminate PTSD-type symptoms. With the heightened stress levels of daily life, most people, if not all, have experienced some level and degree of trauma, so this method works not just for PTSD symptoms, but also for trauma of varying degrees.

Marissa incorporates **somatic and tantric embodiment, breathwork, and sound healing** into the container, which she works intensively with her clients in. These are lifetime-lasting resources and real-life practical skills that can be implemented into daily life moving forward to provide emotional regulation and equilibrium.

The modalities that Marissa offers have proven results and have been combined to maximise the results and provide long-lasting benefits and transformations.

Each element works differently but also in conjunction with each other to accelerate and expedite the results and empower the client to be able to implement these resources and tools into other areas of their life.

Marissa loves working with her clients, but she also loves to see them empowered and ready to move on from whatever has been holding them back.

Marissa is the transformational consultant for those ready to reclaim inner freedom, step into living life on their own terms, take action and do the work to make lasting and deep changes, are ready to uplevel and elevate their life, want to achieve true transformations, and realign with their souls' purpose while aligning to their own unique authenticity and sovereignty.

If you are ready to move through your current plateau and elevate your life – Marissa is the transformational consultant for you!

Marissa is the solution for those who have tried everything but are still not where they want to be. Marissa helps to access your inner wisdom and infinite potential to be empowered to make changes and gain a deeper insight into yourself and your life. What clients come to see Marissa for and what they leave with is far more than they ever expected. If you are ready to do the inner work and be guided and supported along the journey, Marissa is here to help!

With a wealth of knowledge and experience, Marissa is the go-to for expert advice, insights, mindset, motivation, and inspiration. Marissa can tap into and access deeper parts of yourself and have an acute level of understanding of the "why" of people, their behaviours, motivators, and how to achieve lasting levels of transformation.

The areas of expertise Marissa specialises in are:

- Abundance mindset and strategies
- Addictions
- Athletes / Sports performance
- Birth / Conception / Fertility
- Breaking ancestral trauma and generational bonds
- Business Owners – increase success, move to higher levels of performance
- Confidence
- Financial – sabotages and wealth increases
- Healing past trauma
- Health Issues
- Imposter syndrome
- Insomnia
- Life Purpose
- Motivational mindset/ Procrastination
- Relationships
- Self-Esteem / Self-Value / Self-Worth
- Sexual addictions / Disorders / Dysfunctions
- Stress
- Success Strategies

- Weight

If this work sounds like something you need in your life and you are ready to elevate, then please book a free discovery call and let's connect to get you started on your transformation journey.

To help as many people as possible, Marissa has her first book, ***Elevate; Make Change Easy to Transform Your Life***. This book is filled with practical insights, tools and techniques to help you transform your life and move from where you are to where you want to be.

ORDER ELEVATE BOOK

BOOK FREE DISCOVERY CALL

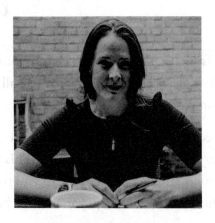

Victoria Stakelum

The Success Smith
Chief Mindset Coach

https://www.linkedin.com/in/victoriastakelum/
https://www.facebook.com/groups/successcollective
https://www.instagram.com/thesuccesssmith/
https://thesuccesssmith.com/
https://getsuccess.scoreapp.com/

Dr Victoria Stakelum is a multi-award winning psychologist and NLP Master Coach – she specialises in how to harness the power of your subconscious mind so you can create success on your own terms.

Victoria's broad and unique toolkit spans energy work, emotional healing, mindset and manifestation.

Underlying all of her methods is a belief that in order to Succeed, you must first Heal. Victoria has supported hundreds of clients to release the negative emotions and limiting beliefs that keep them in procrastination, struggle and unmanifested potential. She helps people heal their self-worth and confidence wounds and develop the skillset and mindset to achieve fulfilment and success in relationships, business and life and wellbeing.

Beneath the Surface:
Why Lasting Change Starts with Rewriting Your Subconscious Script

By Victoria Stakelum

In this chapter I will share the pivotal moment in my wellness journey that resolved a lifetime of difficulty around weight and body image.

My Story: A Lifetime of Struggle

I spent decades locked in a battle with my weight and body image. I can vividly recall the countless times I started a new fitness regime, filled with enthusiasm and determination, only to fall off the wagon within a month. My relationship with food was also tumultuous, marked by emotional and secretive eating that left me feeling out of control, stuffed and then embarrassed and ashamed. My weight fluctuated constantly as I cycled through periods of being the 'good girl'—the one who had it all together—only to crash into weeks of binging on chocolate and feeling completely demotivated around exercise. Much of my life revolved around this body image obsession. I would often be talking or thinking about ways to lose weight or tone up. I was intensely focused on how I looked, often feeling paranoid about quite normal body stuff like the feeling of an elasticated waist pinching into my skin—I hated the feeling of anything ever 'bulging' in any way and was deeply insecure and defensive.

For years, this pattern defined my life. I was caught in an exhausting cycle of self-criticism, shame, and frustration. I desperately wanted to change, but every time I tried, I found myself back at square one, disheartened and defeated.

The funny thing was, by most people's standards, I looked quite normal. I never really went above a UK size 14 (US size 8). While I struggled to commit to a long-term exercise routine, I was almost always engaged in some form of physical activity—whether it was yoga, Zumba, running, kickboxing, or gym classes. I would spend a few weeks or months enjoying one activity before becoming bored, demotivated, or finding excuses to stop. It could be several months before I discovered something new that felt engaging enough to stick with. Whenever I was 'off the wagon', my self-worth would plummet.

Despite these struggles, I had a very successful career. I was a high-profile corporate leader, and my identity as a successful woman in business motivated me to 'look the part'. Being so visible meant it wouldn't do to be bulging over my waistline or looking puffy or heavy. This professional identity helped me maintain a level of discipline, but it always felt like an exhausting 'pressure-driven' effort to keep up appearances as the woman who 'had it all'. During the lockdown of 2020, when, like so many others, I decided to leave that corporate career, the motivation to stay slim and healthy came crashing down along with the leadership identity that had been propping it up. The fragile nature of my motivation around healthy eating and movement was highlighted. And it wasn't until I dug much deeper and further back into my personal story that I found sustainable change.

It was in my mid-forties that I had the simple yet profound realization that finally changed everything and brought me to a place I never thought I would be: of peace, balance, and health. Today, I have a completely healthy relationship with both exercise and food. I'm in the best shape of my life, and I'm able to indulge in treats without spiralling into unhealthy behaviours. So, what changed? How did I, after decades of struggle, finally break free from the chains that bound me?

Turning Point: My Subconscious Narrative

Throughout my years of struggle, I carried a story with me—just at the edge of my awareness—one that I repeated so often it became a part of my identity. This story was not one I was aware I was telling most of the time, but it seemed to become stronger the more I engaged in my struggle with weight and health. It was this:

"I was an obese child."

It would pop out of my mouth, somewhere between an excuse, an explanation or even a way to receive a compliment in the form of "Oh, really? You'd never know."

This narrative was so deeply ingrained that it seemed like an unquestionable truth. Even my husband noticed how frequently I would bring it up, sometimes wondering why I clung to it so tightly.

As a psychologist, hypnosis practitioner, and NLP master practitioner, I have spent years learning about the mind, emotions, and the power of personal development. Yet, it wasn't until I participated in a particular exercise that my own story was challenged in a way I hadn't expected.

During a training program, we were encouraged to connect with our inner child. The exercise involved finding a photograph of ourselves from childhood and sending loving thoughts to that child. As I flipped through the pages of my photo album, a gift from my mother on my 30th birthday, I searched for a picture that resonated with me. What I discovered in those photographs was nothing short of astonishing.

I had never been obese.

In fact, throughout my early childhood, I had been lean, active, and full of energy. I remembered doing gymnastics and ballet, always moving and enjoying my body. It wasn't until I reached the age of ten or eleven that I became a bit chubby, and even then, it was a far cry from the image I had held onto for so long. By fourteen, I was slim again—though by that time, I was struggling with an unhealthy self-image as my story of being too fat, unworthy, and unlovable had begun to take root, leading to extreme measures like starving myself and purging in a misguided attempt to control my weight and feel slim and attractive.

Looking back through those photos, I realized that the story I had been telling myself—and anyone who would listen—was simply untrue. I hadn't been an obese child. I had simply had a few chubby years, which somehow had led to a decision that I was destined to struggle with my weight and health forever more. I had created a narrative that didn't align with reality. But this narrative had become my very identity and had been shaping my life in profound and limiting ways.

The moment I saw the truth in those photographs, everything changed. I let go of the story that had held me back for so long, and in doing so, something extraordinary happened. Over the next six months, I lost over 6 kg, effortlessly, and my relationship with exercise and food was transformed.

Exercise, which had always been a trigger for fear, insecurity, and punishing levels of effort and competitiveness, became something I enjoyed. The negative emotions that once plagued my workouts vanished. I started gravitating toward healthier foods, not because I felt I had to, but because I genuinely wanted to. The need to binge or eat in secret disappeared, replaced by a sense of balance and ease. My transformation wasn't just physical—it was emotional, psychological, and deeply personal.

The Power of Identity and Self-Image

How did this transformation happen so quickly, after years of struggle? The answer lies in the power of identity and self-image.

You see, our beliefs about ourselves—our identity—are the driving force behind our behaviours. If you believe, deep down, that you're meant to struggle with your weight, that you're not someone who can be slim, strong, and healthy, then no matter how hard you try to change, your efforts will be undermined by that underlying belief.

One of my hypnotherapy trainers, Sian Hill, explains this beautifully in her book *Activate your RAS.*[1] She said that when we work consciously through effort and willpower, it's like rowing a boat on the surface of the water. We might row with all our might in the direction we want to go, but beneath the water, attached to the boat by a rope, is a submarine. That submarine represents our self-identity, beliefs, values, and the narratives we carry deep within us. If those unconscious forces are pushing us in a different direction, it doesn't matter how hard we row— we'll either move very slowly or drift off course entirely.

For years, my story—"I was an obese child"—was that submarine, pulling me away from the health and well-being I so desperately wanted. Letting go of that story was like cutting the rope. Suddenly, I didn't have to struggle to move in the direction I wanted to go. I barely had to row, and I made rapid progress toward my goals.

This experience taught me a crucial lesson: If you want to change your behaviour, you have to start by clearing out those identity stories you have accumulated. When you let go of the limiting beliefs that are holding you back, you unlock the ability to make positive changes effortlessly. It's not about using more willpower or trying harder. It's about aligning your self-image with the person you want to become.

From Darkness to Light: Yasmine's Transformation

Let me share with you the story of Yasmine, a client who came to me not for weight loss, but to heal from deep issues of self-esteem and anxiety. Yasmine had endured a traumatic childhood, which left her carrying heavy emotional baggage well into her adult life. When we first met, she was single, depressed, and anxious, trapped in a cycle of negativity that seemed impossible to break.

Our work together focused on releasing negative emotions and limiting beliefs that had been holding her back. We didn't focus on her weight;

---

[1] *Hill, Sian. Activate Your RAS: The Science of Creating Your Reality.* Self-published, 2023. Available at: https://amzn.to/481dXoU.

instead, we addressed the deep-seated pain and trauma that shaped her identity and self-worth.

As Yasmine began to shed these limiting beliefs, something extraordinary happened. Without consciously trying, she started to lose weight. Her body was no longer holding on to the physical manifestation of the emotional weight she had carried for so long. As she continued to heal, she transformed—not just physically, but emotionally and mentally. Today, Yasmine is engaged to be married, radiates confidence, and is at a healthy weight. She is a shining example of how addressing the subconscious stories and emotions we carry can lead to profound changes in all areas of life.

High-Impact Actionable Steps to Unlock Your Journey

Now that you understand the power of identity and self-image, it's time to take action. Here are some high-impact steps you can start taking today to begin your journey toward releasing the subconscious blocks that make behaviour change so challenging.

Step 1: Identify and Challenge Your Current Beliefs

The first step to changing your identity is to uncover the stories and beliefs that are keeping you stuck. Take some time to reflect on the messages you hold about yourself in relation to your weight, health, and body image. What do you tell yourself about your ability to change? Do you believe that you're destined to struggle with your weight? Do you secretly think that you don't deserve to be slim, healthy, and strong?

Write down these beliefs and examine them closely. Ask yourself where they came from. Are they really true, or are they based on past experiences or the opinions of others? Challenge these beliefs by looking for evidence that contradicts them. For example, if you believe that you've always struggled with your weight, find moments in your life when that wasn't true—just like I did with my childhood photos.

Step 2: Reframe Your Identity

Once you've identified your limiting beliefs, it's time to start reframing your identity. Begin by asking yourself, "If I were the person I wanted to be, what story would I be telling?" Imagine the version of yourself who has already achieved the health and well-being you desire. What does she believe about herself? How does she speak to herself? What habits and behaviours come naturally to her?

Start living into that identity today. Visualize yourself as that person, embodying her confidence, strength, and self-love. Write affirmations that reinforce this new identity, and repeat them daily. The more you align your thoughts and actions with your desired identity, the more your behaviours will start to change naturally.

Step 3: Create Space Between Emotion and Action

Many of us turn to food to meet emotional needs, whether it's comfort, love, or stress relief. One of the most powerful tools you can use to break this pattern is to create space between the emotion and the action.

The next time you find yourself reaching for an unhealthy snack, pause. Take a deep breath and ask yourself, "What am I really feeling right now? What need am I trying to meet with this food?" By bringing awareness to your emotions, you can choose a different response. Instead of automatically eating, consider other ways to meet your emotional needs. You might call a friend, go for a walk, do some yoga, or even just sit with your feelings and breathe through them.

If you still decide to eat the food, do so mindfully and without judgment. Allow yourself to enjoy it, knowing that it's a conscious choice rather than an unconscious reaction.

Step 4: Practice Self-Compassion

One of the biggest barriers to change is the harsh inner critic that many of us carry. This voice tells us we're not good enough, that we'll never change, that we don't deserve to be healthy or happy. But here's the truth: Lasting change doesn't come from self-criticism. It comes from self-compassion.

Start treating yourself with the same kindness and understanding you would offer a close friend. When you make a mistake or fall back into old habits, don't beat yourself up. Instead, speak to yourself with love and encouragement. Remind yourself that change is a process, and it's okay to take small steps forward. The more you practice self-compassion, the easier it will be to sustain the changes you're making.

Begin Your Journey Today

You have the power to transform your life, just as I did. It starts with letting go of the stories that no longer serve you and embracing the identity of the person you want to become. The steps I've shared with you are just the beginning of your journey.

If you're ready to take the next step and would like some support, I'm here to help. Whether you're struggling with weight, body image, or any other aspect of your health and well-being, I invite you to reach out to me for a discussion. Together, we can explore the subconscious blocks that are holding you back and create a plan to help you move forward with confidence and ease.

You don't have to do this alone. Change is possible, and it can happen more quickly and effortlessly than you ever imagined. Let's embark on this journey together and unleash the full potential of the strong, healthy, and empowered woman within you.

Contact me at victoria@thesuccesssmith.com or
visit https://thesuccesssmith.com for more information.

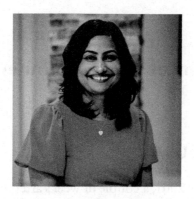

Shraddha Chandwadkar

Self Esteem & Mindfulness Coach

www.linkedin.com/in/shraddhachandwadkar
https://www.facebook.com/people/Luminous-
LifeLabs/61558085485911/
https://www.instagram.com/luminouslifelabs/
https://shraddhachandwadkar.com/

Shraddha Chandwadkar is a passionate Self-Esteem & Mindfulness coach who empowers and illuminates the lives of women and children. Her coaching sessions, workshops & mini-retreats focus on practical strategies to improve self-image, overcome self-doubt, and develop a positive mindset. They also include mindfulness techniques that help in stress management and self-care. When not coaching, Shraddha enjoys writing on topics related to self-esteem, mindfulness, teaching Reiki, and volunteering as an executive program director in a health and wellness non-profit. She recently received the silver 'President Volunteer Service Award' acknowledging her service towards bringing awareness in Mindfulness and Yoga practices. Shraddha is a mother of two teens and three cats. She is also a spiritual seeker who loves to spend quality time in meditative & contemplative practices. An Engineer by education, Shraddha has an MS, Computer Engineering, from NC State University USA and BE in Electronics Engineering from Pune, India.

Beyond Medicine:
A Testimony of Faith and Inner Resilience

By Shraddha Chandwadkar

Welcome to the USA

On December 18th 2001, a couple of weeks after my wedding, I landed on American soil at Raleigh Durham airport in North Carolina with my dear husband. My husband's cousin gave us a ride from the airport. We visited her home for dinner. As soon as we entered her house, my husband whispered in my ears, "Our home is not so big. It is going to be different!" I smiled. Ours was an arranged marriage. We had met in person for only a couple of days before marriage. We had a one-year courtship period. He was in the USA, and I was in India. I honestly was not at all worrying about the home I would be living in. After dinner, my cousin-in-law dropped us at our apartment in Morrisville.

The drive back to our apartment was pitch dark, with hardly any residential places around and deer and tall trees on the way. It felt like an enchanted town. I was used to streets bustling with activity and a lot of noise and air pollution in India. I was in a sense of wonder, observing the natural beauty in Morrisville, the tall trees, and the deer on the roads. It was like a fairy tale. We entered my husband's rental apartment. It was a clean apartment with fresh new paint. Coming to the USA was a dream that had become a reality. Didn't know what was in store for me and how my life would unfold in the following years.

Sunshine Days

I was on a dependent H4 visa during the early years of marriage. At the time, it was prohibited to work on that visa. I have my bachelor's degree in Electronics Engineering from Pune, India. I did not want to stay at home all day. My husband suggested I take the GRE and pursue my master's at NC State University after I become eligible for in-state tuition. While studying for the GRE, I took a few courses at Durham Technical Community College to keep myself active. This helped me to make new friends as well. Some were married immigrants like me, while others were in their teens. It was fun to be back at school. I did not get a good verbal score on my first attempt at the GRE, so I decided to appear for the GRE again. I then applied for a master's in Computer Science program at the Computer Science department at NC State University. My application was rejected. They asked me to apply to the Computer Engineering program in the Computer Engineering department. I followed their directions. A few days later, I received a call from the office staff from the Computer Engineering department. The lady asked me to come and meet the Head of the department at his office. While driving to the university, the radio was full on. The song that was playing on the radio was, "It's a sunshine day." I was full of hope and in an incredibly happy state that day.

When I entered the office, the Head of the department told me that my GRE score wasn't up to the mark, however, he wanted to give me a chance. He asked me to take a summer course, and based on my performance, he would decide if I would be admitted in the fall or not. He was looking for an A on the course. I took the course Architecture of Parallel Computers, which was quite difficult and managed to get a B. Although I badly wanted an A, I was not dejected. I was, in fact, happy I got a B on a difficult course, which meant I understood it. I decided to meet the Head of the department and let him know that I had taken the course but didn't do as well. I also asked my professor if he would recommend me. Which he gladly did. To my surprise, the Head of the department decided to admit me, and the journey toward a master's in computer engineering began in Fall 2003.

Nausea

One month into my master's, I was driving to the university, and at the traffic light, I felt very dizzy. I had intense nausea. I stopped the car and called my husband. Another person passing by stopped his car and waited with me until my husband arrived at the scene.

The nausea continued for days. We finally decided that I should see a gastroenterologist. The doctor thought I was dehydrated. So, he kept me on IV fluids for a day in the hospital. He also asked me to be on a liquid diet for a month and gave me suppositories. I followed a liquid diet that didn't take the nausea away. I was losing a lot of weight and couldn't sleep on an empty stomach. He ran a few tests on me, including an endoscopy. Everything seemed normal. My pregnancy test was also negative. After the endoscopy, the doctor noticed that my stomach and intestine movements were a bit slower. For the intestine movements, he prescribed a medicine called Reglan and also sleep medication as I had lost my sleep due to less nourishment.

When I took the first dose of Reglan, I felt something odd in my mouth. I ignored it. The next day I took a second dose, and my tongue started falling out of the mouth on its own, and the jaw was also opening on its own. I had lost control over it. In medical terms, this is called dystonia. I did not know at the time what was happening to me. I was new to the country, married for barely one and a half years, and I never had such an experience before. It was scary. My husband took me to urgent care. The urgent care doctor checked my reflexes and he couldn't understand what was wrong. A lady who was sitting in the waiting area started reading prayers for me, looking at my condition. The urgent care doctor asked us to rush to the ER. On that day, the ER was very crowded. We had to wait for six hours before they took me in. While we were waiting in the lobby, my husband was requesting the nurses passing by to take me in as he couldn't see my condition. My jaw was opening wide and it had started to hurt. We were also scared that the condition would worsen. One of the nurses sternly replied, "She is not going to die! We have heart patients here we need to take care of first." We were helpless. However, after she said that, I accepted the fact that I was not going to die. I would be absolutely alright. Even though physically I was going through pain and shock, mentally, I was somewhat at ease. I still was not sure if my jaw would be back in position, the tongue in, and if I would get the control back. I had thoughts of paralysis, too. However, I decided to not be affected too much by them. Once the doctor took me in, he gave me a shot of Benadryl and some medication, and within 30 minutes, the dystonia subsided.

I was still in a state of shock, but happy that everything was back to normal. I invited my dear friends to sleep at our home that night. When I look back at this, I laugh at myself for being kind of childish. However, I am grateful for the empathy shown by my friends who came to our home and stayed with us for a night. It was very comforting, and I am very grateful for their kind heart. They never said, "Why are you being so childish? Grow up!" Instead, they came and gave me a hug, and I could feel that they genuinely cared for my well-being.

The actual issue was nausea, though, and not dystonia. Dystonia was a side effect of medication that was given to help with intestine movements. Since I was allergic to Reglan, I could not take that medicine. I had a feeling to stop all medication and take control back in my hand. Not just Reglan but also the sleeping pills, too, as I thought they were making me feel weird, and I had weird thoughts. Instead of being on a liquid diet, I started eating a little bit more. I decided to drink Ensure Plus, too, to gain weight. It took a few months for the nausea to go away on its own. My body was very weak, and I was very skinny then. I had dropped most courses from my master's first-semester schedule but decided to keep one, which was relatively easy, and I was doing well. In December, during Christmas break, I visited my parents in India and consulted my aunt, who is a gynecologist. She asked me to take vitamins and eat all regular food. I did so slowly and steadily, and I was back to feeling normal. I came back to the US and enrolled in a full semester workload. It had taken about 5 months to be completely ok without feeling malnourished and weak.

Turning Point

This incident had shaken my core. I was looking for answers. I started searching for alternative healing methods. I love the internet for this! I enrolled myself in the Reiki level 1 certification course. Reiki is a Japanese healing technique. The Reiki teacher was very experienced and intuitive. She was a hypnotherapist and Reiki Master. Taking Reiki classes with her opened my channels. I started to understand that I was very analytical, and I needed to rest my thoughts and focus on my inner core. As soon as I surrendered my doubts, I began to learn more deeply. After finishing my Reiki level 1 and 2, and my master's certification, my teacher asked me to attend a body, mind, and spirit expo at Raleigh fairgrounds. She said, "You will find many interesting things to learn there, and it will open you up to a whole new world." I followed her recommendation. The following weekend I visited the expo.

The expo was full of alternative healing methods, psychic readers, aura readers, and astrologers. I met Quantum Touch healing teachers at the expo. I was inquisitive to learn more so I signed up for the level 1 course. I continued to practice Reiki and Quantum Touch with my friends and family. It gave me a great sense of joy to practice these alternative healing modalities. My Quantum Touch teachers requested to stay with us for one weekend as their flight to California was from Raleigh Durham Airport, which was close to our home. During their stay, they shared a lot of information on raw food consumption, green juices, supplements, etc. For the next year or so, we decided to follow a mostly raw diet, at least for one meal. For breakfast, we drank green smoothies. It was the most healthy period of my life.

Little did I know then that I was on a spiritual path, and all these incidents were happening for me to turn more and more inwards. I met many spiritual masters on the path. The one that helped me change my thought patterns and know my true self was the Tejgyan Foundation by Tejguru Sirshree. His system of Wisdom has helped me evolve emotionally and spiritually over the years, and I continue to learn and follow his direction. I also came across the path of kriya yoga through the Kriya Yoga Institute and the master Paramhansa Prajnanananda. Both these spiritual practices complement each other. They have helped me not only in my spiritual progress but overall health and wellness as well.

History Repeats

We moved to the Atlanta suburb in 2011 as my husband decided to change jobs after completing his MBA. The first few years went by, settling into the new home and looking after my young children, who were 1 and 5. In 2014/15, I again experienced a health-related condition. This time, I had eaten a piece of bread and milk for breakfast. As soon as I had it, there was intense burning in my abdomen. The burning sensation was getting worse by the end of the day. I decided to drink cumin water made by boiling a few cumin seeds in water. As soon as I drank the cooled-down cumin water, my burning sensation went away. However, I was not able to eat all the food. I decided to have only boiled vegetables for a week with some cooked rice. I started feeling better, but my weight started dropping drastically. I had reached 90lbs from 125lbs. This is when my husband asked me to go see a doctor. I did visit a gastroenterologist, and he did the endoscopy, found nothing, and blamed it on anxiety. He was not ready to listen to the history of eating bread and the burning sensation, etc. This time once again, after going through all the tests and not being able to pinpoint any issue for too much weight loss, I decided to focus on meditation, gentle yoga, and affirmations taught by my spiritual masters and some that I found in books and YouTube videos. During that time, I also had episodes where

I had to stop the car suddenly due to feeling dizzy, shaking of body, and a lot of burping. The shakiness and burping used to subside after an hour. However, this happened randomly an hour after my meals for over 2.5 years. I was terrified by the experience. Tried cutting down certain foods, but the experience did not subside easily. In this condition, I continued with the meditative, contemplative, and yoga practices. My friend taught me a few hatha yoga exercises for free during that time. All these practices helped me to keep myself in a positive frame of mind and prioritize my body-mind mechanism's health. It took 2.5 years for the issue to subside completely. To gain back the weight, it took more than 6 years. The weight loss did not affect my energy, though. I was continuing all housework and other tasks without any issues. The only thing that was affected was driving as the burping and dizziness happened randomly some days and some days it didn't.

Key Learnings

Through these chapters of my life, I have learned some key pointers in navigating Life and its challenges. I would like to share them with you below.

1. Have Faith: Have immense faith in the Almighty and yourself. Faith will help you rise above every situation in your life.

2. Finding Purpose and Deep Meaning: We have been given birth as an opportunity to look beyond just words. It's important to find the subtle meanings hidden behind the veil of doubt, fear, anger, worry, hate, resentment and jealousy. There is deep meaning hidden in every troublesome situation which helps us go deeper and closer towards our purpose.

3. Unconditional Love: Unconditional love is loving without expecting anything in return. Love yourself and others unconditionally. That is the true road to happiness.

4. Pray: Prayer has answers to everything. Pray daily for everyone.

5. This, Too, Shall Pass: Every situation is temporary. Do not give power to negative thoughts and emotions. Look at them as passing clouds.

6. Be Aware of Internal Guidance: We know exactly what our bodies need. If a body needs a doctor, we will know and will be sent to one.

7. Meditate: Meditation is self-care. Learn to meditate and understand your real Self.

8. Breathwork: Breathing exercises will certainly raise immunity. Kriya yoga came into our lives a year before COVID, and we practiced it daily, and I feel that it has kept us safe.

9. Believe in Yourself: No matter what the situation is, we get through it. The situation is not given to us unless we can handle it.

10. Challenges Are Life's Gifts: Every challenge comes with a gift. The gift to rise above and grow emotionally, mentally, financially, and spiritually. In every situation, recognize these gifts.

New Beginnings

Life has given me ample opportunities to learn, grow, and uplift myself. On the path, several people have helped me in some way or another. And through these experiences, I have found meaning and purpose. From a computer engineer to a patent analyst to a real estate entrepreneur, life has given me a lot. However, the most contentment comes by uplifting and empowering people through my experiential learnings from my spiritual journey and my various personal development certifications like self-esteem coaching, Reiki, mindfulness, emotional intelligence, and emotional freedom technique. My way of giving back to the community is by empowering and illuminating women, children, and teens through self-esteem coaching, mindfulness, self-compassion, and self-care. I facilitate workshops, summer camps, and retreats for children and women. Besides this venture, I also volunteer my time as an executive program director in a health and wellness non-profit. I love to spend my free time in meditative and contemplative practices. I also volunteer in the spiritual organizations close to my heart. I celebrate every moment with gratitude and pray for a better world for one and all. I hope my life learnings will help you navigate your life with a little more ease, hope, faith, and joy. Wishing everyone a healthy and blissful life ahead.

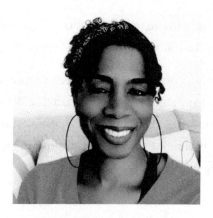

Kimberly Seabrooks

Kim's Health Coaching
Certified Health Coach

https://www.linkedin.com/in/kimberly-seabrooks-90086631/
https://www.facebook.com/kimberly.seabrooks
https://www.instagram.com/kimberlyseabroo/
https://procoach.app/kimberly-seabrooks-2

Kimberly Seabrooks is a Certified Health Coach and a passionate advocate dedicated to empowering women to live their healthiest lives. As the founder of Kim's Health Coaching, a popular YouTube channel, Kimberly has built a strong online community where she shares practical health tips, advice, and inspiring stories. Her content resonates particularly with women in their 40s and 50s, addressing their unique dietary needs during this stage of life.

With a Bachelor's Degree in Business and close to half a decade in the field, Kimberly has dedicated herself to helping women navigate the challenges of aging with grace and vitality. Kimberly's specialization lies in coaching women going through menopause, offering valuable insights and strategies tailored to their unique needs. She emphasizes the importance of adjusting dietary habits to support hormonal changes and maintain optimal health as women age. Through her health coaching program,

Kimberly has positively impacted the lives of numerous women, helping them achieve deep physical and mental well-being.

Recently, Kimberly contributed to the empowering anthology, "Becoming An Unstoppable Woman in Health & Wellness," showcasing her expertise and insights. Through her chapter, she offers invaluable wisdom on how women can harness resilience and overcome the obstacles that come with aging.

The Heart of Health Coaching: My Journey and Passion for Empowering Women

By Kimberly Seabrooks

Introduction

My name is Kimberly Seabrooks, and I am a Certified Health Coach. I have dedicated my life to empowering women to live their healthiest lives. As the founder of Kim's Health Coaching, I have cultivated a strong online community through my popular YouTube channel. This chapter is an exploration of my love for health, my passion for health coaching, and the profound impact this journey has had on my life and the lives of countless women, particularly those in their 40s and 50s.

The Beginning of My Health Journey

My journey into health coaching was not a straight path. With a Bachelor's Degree in Business, I initially embarked on a corporate career. However, my passion for health and wellness was always a constant undercurrent. As I approached my late 30s, I noticed significant changes in my body and health. These changes prompted me to seek knowledge about women's health, particularly around the unique challenges women face as they age.

Through extensive research and personal experience, I realized the critical importance of dietary adjustments and lifestyle changes. This realization ignited a desire to share my newfound knowledge with other women. I wanted to help them navigate the complexities of aging with grace and vitality, just as I was learning to do for myself.

Founding Kim's Health Coaching

In 2019, I founded Kim's Health Coaching with the mission to empower women to take control of their health. The decision to start a

YouTube channel was fueled by my desire to reach as many women as possible. I knew that social media had the power to connect people from all walks of life, and I wanted to create a space where women could find practical health tips, advice, and inspiring stories.

Creating content for Kim's Health Coaching has been one of the most rewarding aspects of my career. I focus on addressing the unique dietary needs of women in their 40s and 50s, a demographic often overlooked in mainstream health advice. Through my videos, I share valuable insights on how to adjust dietary habits to support hormonal changes, maintain optimal health, and improve overall well-being.

Specializing in Menopause Coaching

One of the pivotal moments in my career was when I decided to specialize in coaching women going through menopause. Menopause is a significant life transition that brings about numerous physical and emotional changes. Unfortunately, many women feel unprepared and unsupported during this phase of their lives.

My specialization in menopause coaching allows me to offer tailored strategies and insights to help women manage symptoms and embrace this stage of life. I emphasize the importance of nutrition, exercise, and mindfulness in supporting hormonal balance and overall health. Through my coaching program, I have witnessed the transformative power of personalized guidance and support.

Building a Community of Empowered Women

The most fulfilling aspect of my work is the sense of community that has developed around Kim's Health Coaching. The women who follow my channel and participate in my coaching programs are incredibly supportive of one another. They share their stories, offer encouragement, and celebrate each other's successes.

This community is a testament to the power of connection and shared experiences. Women in their 40s and 50s often face similar challenges, and knowing that they are not alone can be immensely reassuring. The bonds formed within this community extend beyond health and wellness; they foster a sense of belonging and sisterhood.

Contributing to *Resilient: The Power To Get Back Up*

Recently, I had the honor of contributing to the anthology *Resilient: The Power To Get Back Up*. In my chapter, I share my expertise and insights on harnessing resilience and overcoming the obstacles that come with aging. Writing for this anthology was a deeply personal and reflective experience. It allowed me to delve into my journey, the challenges I have faced, and the lessons I have learned along the way.

Resilience is a core theme in my coaching philosophy. Aging can bring about numerous physical and emotional hurdles, but I firmly believe that every woman has the inner strength to overcome them. Through my contribution to *Resilient*, I hope to inspire other women to embrace their resilience and navigate the complexities of aging with confidence and grace.

The Impact of Health Coaching on My Life

Health coaching has not only transformed the lives of the women I work with but also my own life. It has deepened my understanding of health and wellness, strengthened my empathy and compassion, and given me a profound sense of purpose. Helping women achieve deep physical and mental well-being is incredibly rewarding, and it fuels my passion for this work every day.

The Unique Challenges Women Face in Their 40s and 50s

Women in their 40s and 50s face a myriad of unique challenges. Hormonal changes, weight gain, decreased energy levels, and mental health concerns are just a few of the issues that can arise during this stage of life. These challenges are often compounded by societal expectations and the pressures of balancing career, family, and personal well-being.

As a health coach, I strive to address these challenges holistically. I emphasize the importance of listening to one's body, practicing self-compassion, and making informed choices about diet and lifestyle. My approach is rooted in the belief that every woman deserves to feel empowered and in control of her health.

The Importance of Adjusting Dietary Habits

Diet plays a crucial role in managing the symptoms of aging and supporting overall health. For women going through menopause, certain dietary adjustments can make a significant difference. I encourage my clients to focus on nutrient-dense foods that support hormonal balance, bone health, and energy levels.

Incorporating a variety of fruits, vegetables, lean proteins, and healthy fats is essential. Additionally, I advocate for the reduction of processed foods, refined sugars, and excessive caffeine, which can exacerbate symptoms like hot flashes and mood swings. Hydration is another key component, as it helps regulate body temperature and maintain overall well-being.

Exercise and Movement for Optimal Health

Regular exercise is another cornerstone of my health coaching philosophy. Physical activity is not only beneficial for maintaining a healthy weight but also for supporting mental health and emotional well-being. I encourage my clients to find forms of exercise they enjoy, whether it's yoga, walking, dancing, or strength training.

Exercise helps to alleviate stress, improve mood, and enhance sleep quality. For women in their 40s and 50s, it is particularly important to incorporate strength training to support bone density and muscle mass.

Flexibility and balance exercises are also valuable for maintaining mobility and preventing injuries.

Mindfulness and Stress Management

Mindfulness and stress management are integral aspects of my coaching approach. Chronic stress can have detrimental effects on health, particularly during menopause. I teach my clients various mindfulness techniques, such as meditation, deep breathing exercises, and journaling, to help them manage stress and cultivate a sense of calm.

Mindfulness practices not only reduce stress but also enhance self-awareness and emotional resilience. By learning to be present and compassionate with themselves, women can navigate the challenges of aging with greater ease and confidence.

Success Stories and Testimonials

One of the most gratifying aspects of my work is hearing the success stories and testimonials from the women I have coached. These stories are a testament to the transformative power of personalized health coaching. Many of my clients have reported significant improvements in their physical health, mental well-being, and overall quality of life.

For instance, Sarah, a 48-year-old woman going through menopause, struggled with weight gain, low energy levels, and mood swings. Through our coaching sessions, she learned to make dietary adjustments, incorporate regular exercise, and practice mindfulness. Within a few months, Sarah experienced increased energy, improved mood, and a healthier weight. Her story is just one of many that highlight the positive impact of health coaching.

The Future of Kim's Health Coaching

As I look to the future, I am excited about the potential for growth and expansion of Kim's Health Coaching. I plan to continue creating valuable content for my YouTube channel, reaching more women and providing them with the tools and knowledge to live their healthiest lives. Additionally, I am exploring opportunities to develop online courses and workshops to offer more in-depth guidance and support.

My vision is to create a comprehensive platform where women can access a wealth of resources, connect with a supportive community, and receive personalized coaching. I am committed to staying abreast of the latest research and trends in women's health to ensure that my coaching remains relevant and impactful.

Conclusion

In conclusion, my journey as a health coach has been deeply fulfilling and transformative. I am passionate about empowering women to take control of their health and navigate the challenges of aging with grace and vitality. Through Kim's Health Coaching, I have built a strong online community where women can find practical health tips, advice, and inspiring stories.

Specializing in menopause coaching has allowed me to offer valuable insights and strategies tailored to the unique needs of women going through this life transition. Contributing to the anthology *Resilient: The Power To Get Back Up* has further solidified my commitment to helping women harness resilience and overcome obstacles.

The impact of health coaching on my life and the lives of countless women is profound. I am grateful for the opportunity to make a positive difference and look forward to continuing this journey of empowerment and wellness. Thank you for allowing me to share my story and my passion for health coaching. Together, we can achieve deep physical and mental well-being and live our healthiest lives.

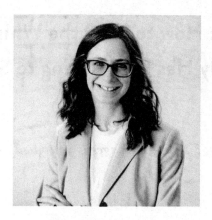

Morgan Staton

Founder and CEO of RestoreHer Wellness
Holistic Wellness Coach

https://www.instagram.com/restoreher_wellness
https://www.restoreherfunctionalwellness.com/
https://calendar.app.google/954CTyeWyvZewuST7

Morgan Staton, MOTRL, FMACP is a former burnt-out mom and entrepreneur, turned holistic wellness coach, after ignoring her body's messages for years and ended up in a crisis state that almost cost her her life. She now uses her background as an occupational therapist and functional medicine practitioner help other busy women make friends with their bodies and get their spark back, so that they can live a life that sets their soul on fire. She believes that there is no one like you on this planet, so your care shouldn't look the exact same as anyone else's. She uses a customized approach of dietary, supplementation, lifestyle, movement, mindset, and nervous system regulation to help women address their concerns at the root cause and get sustainable results of feeling great in their bodies again.

Tuning In: How to Hear the Whispers Your Body Has Been Trying to Send

By Morgan Staton

Are you listening? What messages is your body trying to send to you?

Intro:

When was the last time you felt truly great physically AND mentally within your body?

Not good.

Not alright.

I am talking so great that you would not change a single thing.

Having trouble thinking of the answer?

Feeling kind of sad just thinking about it?

You are not alone. When I came across that question a few years ago after having my first baby, I did not have an answer either. In fact, I was not even sure what "great" felt like in my body. Did anyone actually feel "great"?

Turns out that people who have figured out how to listen to their body when it is sending messages and work with it rather than against it actually felt "great" in their bodies. You see, the thing is, your body and brain are in constant connection with what the body is experiencing on a moment-to-moment basis. However, the brain learns to filter a lot of the messages out because it is not important, or maybe they are important, but we have been ignoring or neglecting them for so long that it no longer recognizes them as important.

Let's do a little experiment: I want you to turn your attention to your right big toe. Really focus on it. What sensations are you experiencing? Now, your brain is so focused on that area that it is consciously sending you signals that have been there the whole time, but I bet that you were not feeling them until I brought it to your attention.

You see, our body is constantly sending signals and messages about everything in and around our body, BUT you have to actually be in tune with your body enough to hear what I call the "small whispers" it is telling us.

My Story:

I, too, used to be so out of tune with my body that I was not even getting the small whispers my body was sending me that something was off until it was screaming at me, and even then, I tried to gaslight myself that it wasn't THAT bad.

I wish I could tell you that I was very good at listening to my body before motherhood, but that would be a lie. The truth is that I probably have never been good at listening to my body. If I am really honest with myself, it was never something that I had learned from the important people around me growing up. I was not taught what rest looks like, how to process emotions in a healthy way, or what it looks like to ask for help and let people in. But that is another story for another book.

Looking back at my life, my body had been sending me signals that something was off for years before I became a mother. I struggled with chronic constipation, to the point that I ended up in ER two separate times for suspected appendicitis. Nope. I was just full of crap. Literally. I also struggled with other issues, including hypothyroidism, low blood sugar and fainting, ovarian cysts the size of softballs and periods that came whenever they wanted.

I never really thought anything of them because a lot of family members were having the same issues. This must have been normal. Just something that happens to women. So, I did what the doctors told me and continued suppressing those messages for years. That is, until my husband and I started trying to get pregnant. I naively thought that it would happen easily for us because it was the experience of other female family members, including my mom, my aunt, and my grandma. It didn't. After 14 months of trying and lots of tests later, I ended up with two new diagnoses: PCOS, also known as Polycystic ovarian syndrome, and Hashimoto's. When I asked what were the steps to resolving those, I was told that I would go back on thyroid medication and that we could start medicated cycles to make getting pregnant easier. Neither of those "solutions" were actually solutions at all, but rather band-aids to underlying issues. I was sick of band-aids.

That was when I started to do my own research. I decided to add about a million supplements into my daily regimen and go dairy- and gluten-free. Basically anything that someone had mentioned on the internet that had worked for them, I did it. At one point, I was taking more than 40 pills a day. My spice cabinet became overloaded with the latest and "greatest" supplements that were going to solve my problem. And we were able to get pregnant, which I was over the moon about. But there were a couple of problems with my "everything but the kitchen sink" approach. The first problem was I was not making dietary, lifestyle, and supplementation changes under the advice of a practitioner. The second problem was that I was still not tuning into my body's signals that it was sending me and approaching them with tailored and targeted thinking to address the root cause of the imbalances in my particular body. And that came back to bite me in the butt when the postpartum period hit.

In the first six weeks of my daughter's life, we all had COVID-19, I was dealing with the aftermath of severe pre-eclampsia with a baby that was born three weeks early, and on top of normal postpartum hormone changes, I had the left half of my thyroid removed. Talk about a chaotic time.

Also, in that time, within about six weeks of delivering, I had returned to my pre-baby weight and was actually slightly under where I was when we conceived. I wrote it off as a result of breastfeeding. I started a new job and went about my life as if nothing was wrong. I continued to lose weight over the next several months and also started to develop severe brain fog and fatigue. I, again, wrote it off as part of motherhood to a baby who did not believe in sleep. I kept ignoring what my body was yelling to me that something was not right.

It was not until my weight continued to drop to 104 pounds, a weight I had not been at since middle school, and my arms and legs started to go numb intermittently, that I finally started to tune into what my body was trying to tell me. But at that point, those "whispers" had become so prominent that they were essentially b*tch slapping me in the face and yelling, "WAKE UP AND DO SOMETHING ABOUT THIS." That started a cascade of events that included thousands of dollars worth of testing, 10 specialists on my team, my ability to be a mother to my child and do my job limited, and no answers or plan for treatment. My team essentially told me, "We know something is wrong, but we can not exactly pinpoint what it is, so we can not do anything at this time. We are really sorry, and we will see you in six months."

That was a turning point for me. The quality of life I was experiencing was not something that I was willing to live with for the rest of my life, and if my team could not find the answers, I was going to have to search myself to find them. That started a long and tenuous healing process that was much more than just shoving supplements into my mouth and praying for the best. I really had to tune into my body. I had to get to know my nervous system, my "tells" when my body was overextended, and what changes my particular body needed. I had to figure out how to ask for help, how to be honest with myself and my husband about how I was feeling (because up until that point, I had been in somewhat of a denial and was shielding him from all the physical and mental pain I was experiencing). I also had to figure out what my capacity for change was for dietary and lifestyle changes, and what movement and mindset shifts I needed to make to fully serve my body in the best way possible.

Slowly, I clawed my way out of what I can only describe as hell. I started to gain more energy. My brain fog decreased. My arms and legs stopped going numb. My weight loss stabilized and I slowly started to gain weight back to a healthier weight for my body. All without taking a million supplements a day. Don't get me wrong, I definitely still took supplements, but this time the supplements were a compliment to what my body was actually asking for, as well as the other very intentional changes I had been making slowly over time.

When I look back on that time now, a couple of thoughts come to mind:

1. Things were SO much worse than I allowed myself to believe for so long.

2. I wish I had tuned into my body sooner, and feel after neglecting my body, mind, and soul for so long.

3. I am thankful for all that I went through because it led me down the path toward becoming a functional medicine practitioner and holistic wellness coach and now allows me to deeply support other busy women in making friends with their bodies and getting their spark back so that they can live a life that sets their soul on fire.

Common things your body may be trying to tell you

Maybe reading my story felt like I was in your brain telling yours. Or maybe it's the same song but a different instrument, as they say, meaning the exact experience may not be the same, but the essence of ignoring your body and having things that you would like to change but you have been dismissed or brushed off is the same.

Maybe you are reading this and are thinking to yourself: But what can the messages mean?

I want to break down some root causes for things women typically experience so that you are not running around like a chicken with your head cut off trying to find solutions to a problem you can't even put a name to.

Let's talk about physical tension first. As women, we often hold tension in several areas of our body that are actually related to emotional things going on, here is what that can mean:

- Shoulders: lots on your mind, taking on too much.
- Chest: chronic stress/fight or flight, fear of failing, saying or doing the wrong thing
- Stomach: unprocessed emotions about circumstances, either past or present
- Back: lack of support physically, emotionally, and/or financially
- Pelvis: lack of safety, nervous system dysregulation, abandonment, criticism from yourself or others

I also want to touch on some conditions or sensations that are very common but not normal. These can be a sign that your body needs some additional support:

- Difficulty falling or staying asleep
- Digestive problems (constipation, diarrhea, bloating, heartburn, nausea, etc.)
- Mood swings
- Headaches
- Unexplained weight gain or loss
- Irregular, heavy, or painful periods
- Decreased libido
- Skin changes (rashes, acne, dry skin, etc.)
- Brain fog, difficulty concentrating or remembering
- Autoimmune conditions
- Intense sugar or salt cravings

- Getting sick more frequently

You may have one of these things or all of them. Either way, these are all signals your body is sending you that it needs additional support in a specific area.

Strategies for tuning into your body's messages

Maybe you have read through this chapter and thought to yourself: I don't even know what my body is trying to tell me.

Don't feel bad about that. You are not alone. When you have gotten so good at ignoring the signals, it can be hard to start to listen. Because of that, I want to leave you with a reflection exercise that you can do. Ideally, if you are having trouble connecting with your body, I recommend doing it at least daily, but you can do it as often or as little as you feel like. It shouldn't take more than a couple of minutes out of your day. For my ladies who are thinking, "I can not add another thing into my day," I encourage you to pair this exercise with going to the bathroom because you HAVE to do that at some point in the day, or your bladder is going to be VERY unhappy with you. You can think through these questions mentally or journal about them if that feels more aligned with you.

Don't overthink this exercise, and approach it from a place of curiosity. There is no wrong or right answer. Whatever comes to mind is right for you in the moment. It may change each time you do it, even if you do it multiple times a day. It also may stay the same. Both are okay! If you are really struggling with connecting, try pretending your body is someone else's and that you are asking these questions from an outside perspective.

Here are the questions you should ask yourself:

1. Start to scan your body slowly from head to toe, what sensations are you experiencing?

2. Are there areas or sensations that are more prominent for you? Can you try to describe those sensations with a color, shape, or visual picture? For example: a ball in the throat or an elephant sitting on my head?

3. Sometimes we hold things for other people. Ask, "Is this mine to hold, or am I holding it for someone else? If you are holding it for someone else, try to let it go and see if that sensation dissipates.

4. Ask yourself the following three questions: What does my body need? What does my mind need? What does my soul need? The answers may be different, and even contradictory, from each other. That is okay. The important thing is to notice what is coming up and see how you can incorporate that answer into your day to better serve your body, mind, and soul.

What's next?

If this chapter felt like I was speaking to your soul, I would love to connect and hear your biggest takeaway. If you find that you are wanting more support, here are some options to start or continue this journey:

1. Listen to my podcast: *The Ignited Woman,* wherever podcasts are available.

2. Request a complimentary Whole Body Wellness Assessment and review. I will be able to tell you the exact areas where your body needs additional support and provide individualized recommendations so that you can save time and money and avoid "everything but the kitchen sink" to feel great in your body both physically and mentally.

3. Instagram: @Restoreher_wellness

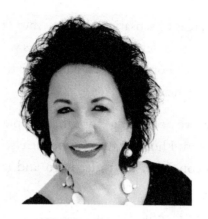

Sherry Anshara

QuantumPathic Inc and Anshara Institute
Founder & President

https://www.linkedin.com/in/sherryanshara/
https://www.facebook.com/sherryanshara
https://www.instagram.com/sherryansharaofficial/
https://sherryanshara.com/
https://ansharainstitute.org

Sherry Anshara is an international bestselling author, professional speaker, and former radio host of "Conscious Healing." She is also the host of the podcast 'The Quantum Truth' and the 'Medical Intuitive Channel' on Roku TV. As a contributing writer to national and international publications, Sherry shares her insights on the Anshara Method of Accelerated Healing & Abundance and overall wellness.

With over 31 years of experience as a Medical Intuitive and Success Coach, Sherry developed the Anshara AHA! Method®, a groundbreaking approach to healing that focuses on accessing Cellular Memories. This method addresses the root causes of various symptoms—whether mental, physical, emotional, spiritual, or financial—by eliminating limitations, negative thought patterns, and toxic behaviors.

Sherry's journey began with her own healing, using the Anshara Method to recover from severe injuries, including a broken back, neck, and head trauma. Her success led her to assist thousands of people worldwide in healing their bodies and lives from illness, disease, and trauma.

At the Anshara Institute of Accelerated Healing, Sherry trains facilitators and practitioners to use her method, amplifying its impact and helping more individuals achieve health, wellness, and abundance in every area of their lives.

An Inner Journey of Self-Discovery Within!

By Sherry Anshara

1991, an extraordinary experience changed my life. In retrospect, although it didn't appear this way at the time, this experience that resulted in my death brought me to life! Though a Near Death Experience can appear unusual, strange and even astonishing, there are living deaths that happen. Death doesn't always mean dead! Death can mean a change, a shift, and/or a completion of some kind.

The death of a relationship, the death of a way of life, the death of something. In my case, death really occurred. Yet, through this event, deep within me an expected and even astonishing change occurred that swept through me from my deepest core of knowledge within me.

Not to be dramatic about this event, but this experience did not support what you might think is an immediate change in my life. Of course, an immediate shift occurred. Yet it became an ongoing process, that I would eventually recognize as a "progress process" that shifted, changed the very essence of me from my deepest sense of me from the inside out! Yes, it is a progressive process. The Isness is in the moment.

"STAY FOCUSED, STAY OUT OF THE DUALITY TIME LOOPS, EMBRACE YOUR CONNECTIONS FROM THE INSIDE OUT, BE IN THE MOMENT, EMBRACE YOUR SELF!!!"

There is so much knowledge gained in a progressive process which I would discover as I progressed. This progression took place, sometimes in immediate changes or shifts, in how I viewed "life". I also began to recognize that this progression had a process to it of viewing life from many different angles and views. The different angles and views actually evolved into what I call NEO, Non-Emotional Observer. This standpoint is completely freeing from any emotional attachments to any dramas or traumas, past, present or recreated in the future!!!

Though I had many fractures in my head and body, very painful, at times worse than others, deep within me, intuitively and sometimes not so clear, I began to see and experience changes in others. Yes, this progressive process happened, sometimes with me kicking and screaming. Denial is so often connected to defiance. How many times has anyone who experienced life-changing experiences, divorce, loss of any kind, person, job, lifestyle, being alone or rejected reacted in defiance? Surely many of us jumped into survival mode.

Perfectly understandable! Life-changing, life-altering! However, these life-altering, life-changing experiences and situations can turn out to be the most surprising and special life-altering, knowledge-gaining occurrences. In my own personal and professional case, this is what happened.

As I lay in a hospital, with dire predictions for my life, it appeared so scary and threatening. Yet, with the best YET, my life began to evolve in the most remarkable ways. As I lay in this hospital bed, asking my own body, which was in a physical and emotional mess from every view or so it seemed, two words came to me... Cellular Memory! Cellular Memory, what the heck is this? At times, in pain, looking like a mess with these injuries, not even knowing at the time that my brain was out of place within my cranium, bruised, and stitches in my head with very broken areas within my body, these two words coming from the depths within me would change my life and the lives of others.

I didn't know how profound these two words would change my life, but eventually, they would change thousands of lives from their insides to their outside worlds. My body was providing me with answers as I asked my body if there must be something smarter within me; because my head, brain and body were challenged to the max!

Through this inner knowledge from 1991, the following years then gave me a new start in life. With the physical and emotional issues, it became challenging to work, to live the life I had created for my Self. The life as I had known it was not working at all! The challenges, physically, emotionally, mentally, spiritually and financially, affected, effected and "infected" me to the max.

The "infect", though at the time I didn't understand any of the physical and emotional messes I was in, turned out to be the "infect" of belief systems, the B.S. as I call it, which did not support me in those moments of self-doubt, self-judgment and self-confusion. Life was not as it was supposed to be. All that I worked so hard for was going away. In some ways, it almost appeared to me that all these traumatic experiences and events were happening instantly in my brain. Though it was a process, I discovered later I was not in a progressive process of comprehending what was happening to me. I was being "processed" by Belief Systems, the B.S. of what I was told to "think," how I was supposed to be, supposed to do and supposed to have.

The "supposed to" didn't align with me. As I was going through all these discombobulating changes and shifts, soon a discovery inside of me shouted out, look at all the times in your life when life didn't align with me, no matter how much I had or didn't have! Hmmm, Alignment! A very deep connection to the knowledge inside of me. Looking back, not reliving my life, there were so many times at many of my ages and stages of life when I did the "right" things, but inside, there was not an alignment!

WOW! Another very deep recognition of my Self from the inside out. My own clear Cellular Memory caused me to not only get my answers from within me, but to now recognize how to ask questions of my Self. These questions were not based on what was right or wrong with me. These questions were based on what was correct or not correct for me. A huge paradigm shift began to occur within me!

The discovery allowed me to ask clear, pertinent, make-sense questions. My body began to become very connected within me. Clear questions produced clear answers. These questions began to show me this! QUEST at my ION levels made the difference in my life of what I did or didn't do! ION means Cellular. What was happening was a deep connection to my own inner knowledge, my own inner consciousness, that when I asked the questions at my Cellular Levels, the information provided to me, from me was clear, pertinent and my own answers which were full of my own inner Truth!

This technique or progressive process turned into Wordology Is Your Biology, which I then trademarked. But the best is that Wordology is ALL of Our Biology, not just the physical and emotional process through the brain. The words or language are processed through the Clear Cellular Memory Consciousness of your body's knowledge that provides you, me and everyone's best inner NI, Natural Intelligence.

Through my experiences from 1991, it did, in fact, turn out to be an incredible progressive process. However, from an outside view, a total failure occurred for me. I lost everything. Yes, everything. My beautiful home, my savings, even my family and many of my friends! I became homeless in the best way! They told me to shape up and get a job. Do what I was supposed to do!

Little did they know, those moments were the best times of my life, though from an outside view my life did not appear very good. The best times were happening from the inside of me to my outside world. Time didn't appear to be on my side. Yet time became my most valuable friend when, in fact, during all this turmoil, learning about what time is and what it isn't made so many valuable, seemingly awful moments become the best moments of my life.

Knowledge from within came in those moments of clarity and insight. The insights of my own inner vision of how, what, where, when and why in these Non-Self-Judgment moments, the clarity of answers from within me begin to unfold.

With all these physical and emotional dysfunctions from an outside view, from within me came clear, direct and focused answers. Not from the limitations of my left computer brain, the answers came from within me. My Cellular Memory unleashed all this inner knowing and clear knowledge of what my life would be about.

The reasons for being here!!! Did it happen in one moment, an hour, a day, a week? No! In our idea of linear time, it was weeks, months and years and continues to unfold each and every day. The difference now, than in those days after my accident in 1991, is my body knew how to heal itself. Yet my left computer brain was engaging in survival mode for what seemed to be forever.

The forever is what is the ever for? The ever is for being in the moment. The more I stayed in the moment and allowed my Cellular Memory to unfold, the faster my body healed. Though two more Near-Death Experiences would follow, especially the dramatic Third One, they were blessings beyond anything that could be measured in my life.

Laughing many times, with four dramatic head injuries, my brain challenged to the max, the more I knew that something absolutely divine was occurring within me. Through these challenges, the gains were extraordinary. So I asked my Self from time to time, "Why did I have to do these things so dramatically and traumatizing?" Well, the answer was always the same, "You wouldn't listen to Your Self!" What a tough sell! OMG!

Now there is no reason to sell anything to my Self, especially limited Belief Systems, that I identified as B.S. The best part is not losing my sense of humor. There is no doubt about it: my proverbial sense of humor really "saved" me from my limited Self. Humor is the best medicine.

Using laughter, as the core of the best medicine, made me "see" life from a different perspective. Perspective in the core of something provides the facts. Perceptions, on the other side of the coin, are emotional without facts. This view became the first tool that would become part of my Anshara AHA! Method® years later. This view shaped, produced and formed a position for me and eventually for my friends and clients to become NEO!

"PERCEPTIONS ARE THE RECEPTIONS AND DECEPTIONS OF MY CONCEPTIONS!"
—Sherryism

What is NEO? Non-Emotional Observer. A position that provided facts instead of conjectures! Now, without the emotional "attachment" to an experience, situation, event and even relationship, personal and/or professional, a clear view happens. In this clear Non-Emotional Observation, NEO clarity happens. In this clarity, Conscious Choices instead of emotional decisions are made.

The differences are remarkable in establishing your life in the most powerful ways. In this stance as NEO, Non-Emotional Observer, you make clear Conscious Choices, which are flexible and changeable. Through the years of working with my Self first and clients/friends, the practical discovery of how someone creates his or her life through this remarkable tool of NEO made huge differences. The differences showed up in the personal health and personal empowerment of those who have used this first tool.

This tool is part of my own Self-Discovery from within me. The more emotional I got or gave into the emotionality of a situation, event or relationship, the more difficult it was to create and establish my life. The giant AHA is the moment realizing that my Left Computer Brain is the culprit and has always been the problem in my life. The more I became NEO, Non-Emotional Observer, the healthier, the more productive and the more creative my life became.

Life is a Progressive Process. However, from this observer standpoint, when all the emotionality is being "conducted" through the Left Computer Brain, the more Non-Productive life happens. Emotionality caused so many trauma dramas! These trauma dramas use up or waste creativity. They waste life. They take time!

The problem is that without the stance of NEO, Non-Emotional Observer, the trauma dramas get stuck in the Left Computer Brain. As this happens, though the circumstances may appear or seem the same, they are not. What happens is that the Left Computer Brain gets caught up in emotional traumas and dramas and can't discern what time it is.

This is the reason so many repeat the same experiences. Though they appear different because of different times at the core, the emotionality of the triggers fire, and the repetition occurs repeatedly. The words that go along with this: "Why is this always happening to me!" The resonance of these repeated trauma dramas inflicts the resonance of being a "victim."

This victim program is actually defined as Duality. What is Duality? Duality is the two emotional sides of a story, an experience, a trauma drama that is repeated. Again, though the circumstances may appear different at the core, hence this word Duality. Again, what is Duality? Duality means opposition, antagonism, adversary, enemy. Where does this start?

Duality begins with the programming of the Left Computer Brain being disconnected from the Right Computer Brain. In the physicality of the human body, the Left Computer Brain activates the Right Male Side, not gender, that "manifests" what is being created in the outside world from the inside. Only using a half brain is not being the Full Monty of Your Self.

Each side of the brain, when disconnected from the other, is not a full computer working as it is intended to. Your Real Brain is your Heart. The Brain in the head functions as an organizational component. This is how it works when connected. A person, regardless of gender, creates through the Female Left side of the Body using the Right Computer Brain to organize what is being created, the Body implements what is being created, and the Left Computer Brain organizes through the Male Right Side of the Body what you are "manifesting," and through the Heart and through both arms and hands, what you are actualizing in your life.

CREATE, IMPLEMENT, MANIFEST AND
ACTUALIZE: THE FOUR WORDS THAT MEAN
THE 4 STEPS OF BEING THE GOODNESS WITHIN
YOU!!!

THIS IS YOU THROUGH YOUR
CONNECTEDNESS WITHIN YOU. THROUGH
YOUR HEARTNESS IS YOUR CREATIVE
ALLNESS!

As you recognize and Realize with "Real Eyes" who you are from the inside out, connecting to your NI, your Natural Intelligence, is the shift that has been talked about for years and years. This shift actually begins to be Actualized within your own amazing body of Consciousness as you connect with your NI, Natural Intelligence, in your body called your Cellular Memory!

Your Cellular Memory occurs the minute the sperm hits the egg, and you are here. You have "your script in hand," metaphorically speaking through your Cellular Memory. Your Cellular Memory is your inherent knowledge of who you are. In a manner of speaking, your nose knows to be a nose cell, and your toe knows to be a toe cell, or there would be a nail at the end of your nose!!!

Humorously with joy and focus, looking at your body, as you connect to your Cellular Memory, your body remembers how to be healthy, flexible and creative. Your Cellular Memory holds all of your own inner knowledge of you through your Continuum. These Memories at the core of you within your Cells, Molecules, and Particles to the Subatomic Levels of you "remembers" the brilliance of you.

YOU HOLD ALL THE TIMES, EXPERIENCES,
AND YOUR OWN INNER KNOWLEDGE WITHIN
YOU AS A MULTI-DIMENSIONAL PERSON...AN
EXTRAORDINARY HUMAN BEING FROM
WITHIN!

Yes, for sure, there are steps in every process. This "shift" is a Consciousness Shift that is occurring from the inside out. This expands the resonance in your body to be healthy. The best wealth anywhere in the world, regardless of currency, is SELF-HEALTH. This resonance of Self-Health is the best paradigm shift from the inside out!

The tools of NEO, Non-Emotional Observer, connecting to NEL, Non-Emotional Listening, from within Your Self are the dynamics that launch this new paradigm of Self-Connectedness from the inside out! The greatest and most practical applications of this Inner Paradigm Shift change this word "Because" from a word of excuse, that you can't create or do something because of the confines of Duality. Now the word becomes Be-Cause! You are being the cause and causation of what you create and do every moment of your life!

THE GOAL IS TO CREATE, IMPLEMENT, MANIFEST AND ACTUALIZE YOUR LIFE AS YOU CHOOSE TO BE IT!

Time becomes the inner space within you of your creative abilities to launch your life every moment. The more you are "willing" to recognize Your Self as this extraordinary person with unlimited capabilities to determine how you live your life. A significant Key to this shift from your inside out is Self-Trust.

As you begin to trust Your Self, letting go or releasing the limitations taught to you through your Left Computer Brain, this resonance of Trust begins little by little. Then a potential avalanche of creativity can be unleashed from within you.

The greatest role models throughout history had to Trust themselves. These were and are the paradigm shifters who made differences in their own lives and the lives of others. Two paradigm shifters who changed the world were Henry Ford and Barry Gordy.

Without judging them personally and/or professionally, it was through their creativity that paradigm shifts occurred. Contrary to popular beliefs, Henry Ford did not invent cars, his contribution, whether you liked him or not, is the assembly line. This practical application of producing any kind of product changed the world of production. Like in any industry, his assembly line in his time-frame changed the worlds of industry around the world.

Barry Gordy, the founder of Motown, worked on the assembly line at Ford Motor Company. With some so-called failures, to make his seemingly long story short, he changed the music industry. How? By taking the assembly line method and applying it to music. He established an assembly line of putting together music, talent, artists and changed how music was created, implemented, manifested and actualized.

Whether anyone liked, judged or unaware of what these two individuals did, they did it in extraordinary ways. Looking at Duality's idea of black and white, good or bad, right or wrong, even from the Duality standpoint of Color, these two men, one white and one black, changed history.

They were not bound by limitations. Now whether you like them or not, looking at the eras in which they created what they did, they were perfect in their timing. They used the time to their advantage. With all the stuff, called in the moment, and now called history, many people did not believe what they were doing. There was judgment going. Yet so what!

Through their inner abilities and knowledge in times appearing to be challenging, like all times, they provided extraordinary changes and shifts to their industries. Now, in this moment of time, within you, or some reading this chapter, perhaps there is a chapter within you, as a WOMAN who has an idea that might change your world or the world around the world.

There are many women throughout history, so-called ahead of their times, who challenged the Duality Limitation Programs. Their challenges made a difference in their current times and in our times now!

Looking through-out history, how many women were behind the scenes? Who knows the numbers? The point is, NOW in this time-line, let's consider "Her"story and "Her"stories that will be historical in the current moment and create productive and practical shifts and changes.

The Woman or Female is the essence of creativity regardless of gender. The Feminine is the foundation of creativity from the inside out. Accessing this resonance is Healthy and produces Wealth, not just in money but in ways beyond measure. The Wealth of Female Creativity is not about Gender. This is about the core of how everyone creates their lives, their personal and professional lives.

As these practical tools are manifested and actualized, paradigm shifts, yes, shifts, in the plural, begin to occur naturally. These natural actualizations are through this inner shift of Non-Duality Consciousness from within to the outside world. These are the actualizations unlimited of productivity, creativity and efficiency. This is establishing Newness.

What is Newness? Newness is the essence, the spirit, the heart and the core of creating, implementing, manifesting and actualizing something new. Even in the new, it can be based upon something that had previously been actualized. Yet adding a new perspective! Not a repeat of something that doesn't work. The example of Motown in the best ways of the assembly line is Newness in the Music Industry.

Creating changes by taking from the BEST of the past, whenever that is, and applying Practical Applications to life NOW. Using your Intuition with Practical Applications to your life. What is your Intuition? Your intuition is your Natural Innate Ability to discern what is correct for you or not. It has nothing to do with "right" or "wrong" in the Left Brain Programming of Duality. Duality makes everything right and then wrong and then right and then wrong.

Another Key to becoming Non-Duality Conscious and stepping into your NI, your Natural Intelligence, is by integrating both sides of your Computer Brain through Your real brain, Your Heart, the practical magic happens. Your Intuition, which means, "In to 'it' at your 'ion' or Cellular Levels of your Natural Intelligence," opens. The "IT" is your Inner Truth! The Isness of your Inner Truth is your Inner Self. This may seem like a play on words. Well, words can empower you or take your Power Away. Another way to unlimit Your Self is to recognize that Wordology is Your Biology.

"What you say makes your day...and what you can say can make or break someone else's day!" —Sherryism.

Your words, your comments through words, your experiences through words make the differences in your Life. Yes, differences. Having supported and assisted individuals with these tools and not speaking their language at all, with an interpreter, these individuals connected to the core, the origination point or points of the Duality traumas, regardless of their diagnoses, and through these connections to their NI, Natural Intelligence, they were able to discern the dramatic differences between the Cellular Memorizations of the Left Computer Brain and connect to their perfect Cellular Memory. Healing began to occur naturally!

Cellular Memorizations through the Duality Left Computer Brain are all the programs that say: You are not worthy, you have no value, you did this wrong, you can't do something, you are whatever label of confinement or restrictions they produce. This is not productive-producing. This is the result of restricting you from any age or stage of the Duality Programming that makes you less and takes away your own Inner Power!

These practical tools for healing Your Self from the inside out is a Progressive Process. These tools are an inner paradigm shift that is established one step at a time. This occurs in the Space within You of the No-Time. The No-Time is to stop measuring Your Self by a tape measure or yard-stick of what you didn't do or can't do. The words within this place and space of the No-Time is this space of resonance of Conscious Creation. The instant an idea comes from within your Real Brain, Your Heart, you intuitively "comprehend" you are onto something.

That something, a Newness Idea, an Observation of how you are Consciously Choosing to participate personally and professionally in your life, with that Paradigm Shift of inner excitement that you onto something of Newness for you. There are no restrictions or reservations. You become Healthy naturally.

The paradigm shift is happening naturally! Your body recognizes the shifts or changes at your Cellular Levels of YOU! The Progressive Process is Step #1 Neo Non-Emotional Observer, Non-Emotional Listener and connecting to your NI, Your Natural Intelligence within YOU! Your Real Brain, your Heart, recognizes this Natural Shift or Change of resonance from within You!

The Cells, Particles and Molecules to the subatomic level of you throughout your body begin to remember, through your Natural Intelligence, how to heal from within. Then, anything you use, supplements, any type of treatments or meditation, will support and assist your body to be healthy and stay healthy.

One of the most significant changes that occur from the inside out through connecting to your NI, your Natural Intelligence, your Cellular Memory, is that you slow down the aging process. This is the best Anti-Aging process! This is the best perk of getting Non-Duality Conscious in this life! Slow down the aging process! Healthy Cells, Particles and Molecules to your subatomic level talking to each other in whatever system they make up!

Through this Progressive Process of YOU connecting to your Body Non-Emotionally, asking your Body clear Non-Emotional Questions, and listening to your body Non-Emotionally through your Real Brain,

Your Heart, you support and assist Your Self in Self- Healing. Healing is addressing the emotional and physical emotional issues in your tissues at the Cellular Level.

As you have these Conscious Conversations with Your Self through the resonance of your Heart, your body begins inner dialogues within each system of your body. Your body begins to communicate within. Through the Energetic Connections, your body supports itself to be healthy. You can call this healing. You can call this being healthy. You can call this becoming your healthy, vibrant and alive Self!

YOUR SHIFT IN CONSCIOUSNESS BEGINS YOUR OWN ENERGETIC CONNECTEDNESS, REAL CONNECTIONS OF CONVERSATIONS WITHIN THE SYSTEMS OF YOU AND YOUR BODY... THIS IS YOUR PRACTICAL QUANTUM BODY, YOUR OWN QUANTUM PHYSICS IN PRACTICAL ACTIONS!

What is Energy? Energy is a byproduct of you. Though the idea is that everything is energy, what does that mean? Every aspect of you, everything you create in your life, is based upon the release of your energy from the inside out. Energy is the propulsion of movement or non-movement from within you to your outside world.

When your Duality Belief Systems, the limitations affect, effect and infect your Natural Abilities to produce your life, you become limited in everything. This happens again and again through the Duality Programming of your Left Computer Brain. This resonance prevents the connection and connectedness to utilizing your Whole Brain to organize what you are creating, implementing, manifesting and actualizing in your life. Limitations become a way of life. No Judgment. This is how your Energy is drained, depleted and gets stuck. When your energy, which is physical, gets stuck, illness, disease and dysfunction happens. Illness, disease and dysfunction are NOT Natural in any way.

Though the Duality Programming will say it is!

The Conscious Connectedness, when you are willing to be your own Paradigm Shift from the inside out, you will "feel" your own energy as a Bi-Product of YOU and Your unlimited, unrestricted Consciousness. Your Energy is the propulsion mechanism that is natural to your Body.

What you Project through your Natural Energy, when your body is in alignment with YOU and Your Unlimited Connections to all your systems, to all your Cellular Memories, the Cellular Memorizations, the limited programming begins to dissolve within you!

YOU and Your Body become the unlimited Allness of YOU. Through your willingness to be your own Paradigm Shifter, to become unlimited Consciousness, you are in charge of your Health, your best Wealth and create wealth outside or you from within YOU!

YOU TAKE BACK YOUR POWER...YOU BECOME YOU!

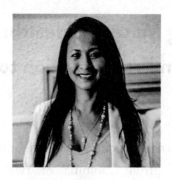

Neliza Patterson

Postpartum Holistic Health and Recovery Practitioner,
Certified Hypnotherapist & Health Coach

https://www.facebook.com/innertranquility.life?mibextid=LQQJ4d
https://www.instagram.com/nelizapatterson/
https://innertranquility.life
https://calendly.com/innertranquility/wellnesscheckin

Neliza Patterson is a devoted mother and a transformative force in maternal wellness. As the founder of Inner Tranquility, a Postpartum Holistic Health and Recovery Practitioner, and a first-time author, Neliza blends professional expertise with personal experience to guide mothers on their unique journeys. Her approach focuses on holistic self-discovery, balancing core values, personal aspirations, and the complexities of motherhood. Passionate about holistic wellness and nutrient-packed superfoods, Neliza specializes in helping moms reprogram their mindset, boost nutrition, and experience the complete essence of motherhood. With a background in the medical field and a personal triumph over Postpartum Depression, she provides compassionate, tailored support, equipping mothers to navigate emotional and physical changes with confidence. Neliza's journey from despair to vitality fuels her mission to å mothers at every stage. Her upcoming #1 bestselling book, "Decoding Baby Blues & Postpartum Struggles," offers crucial insights and strategies to mothers worldwide.

Empowering Maternal Health: Nourishing Wellness from Preconception to Postpartum

By Neliza Patterson

Welcome to your journey of holistic maternal health and wellness. I'm Neliza Patterson, a proud momma of two, founder of Inner Tranquility, a Maternal Health Practitioner, and a first-time author of the upcoming book *Decoding Baby Blues & Postpartum Struggles*. My mission is to empower and nurture mothers through every stage of motherhood with holistic wellness practices and nutrient-packed superfoods. I'm passionate about helping moms reprogram their mindset, boost their nutrition, and thrive in their journey to a more fulfilling motherhood.

With my background as a Registered Diagnostic Cardiac Sonographer and training in Rapid Transformational Therapy and hypnotherapy, I offer a unique blend of expertise and empathy. My goal is to integrate your core values and aspirations with your journey of motherhood, helping you achieve a balanced and fulfilling life.

In this chapter, we'll explore maternal wellness through holistic practices, nutrient-rich superfoods, and practical guidance. We'll navigate your challenges and celebrate your victories, using insights from my transformative journey.

As we begin, I'll share my personal story of transformation and the lessons learned along the way to guide you toward vibrant health and well-being.

Personal Journey

Challenges and transformative moments marked my journey into holistic health and wellness. As a mother, I faced physical, emotional, and mental hurdles that seemed insurmountable at times. It was through these experiences that I discovered the power of holistic healing practices. By addressing the root causes of my challenges rather than just managing symptoms, I found a path to true wellness. This journey has fueled my passion for helping other mothers navigate their paths to health and well-being.

The Challenge

My journey began with one of the most challenging periods of my life. Due to high-risk complications in my pregnancies, caused by age and a rare condition, my world was upended. The difficulties I faced pushed my mental and physical health to their limits. I found myself isolated, overwhelmed by anxiety, and struggling with profound loneliness and self-doubt, which ultimately led to postpartum depression (PPD).

The Turning Point

The turning point in my journey came during an incredibly challenging time. After my husband decided to separate and move out of the house, I was left to manage the household and care for my two young boys on my own. The weight of this upheaval, combined with mounting physical issues that I was not fully aware of, was overwhelming.

One pivotal moment while driving with my boys stands out vividly. The stress and pressure of trying to stay strong and maintain a semblance of normalcy had taken its toll. During that drive, I experienced a blackout and found myself in an unfamiliar place, unable to recall how I had even arrived there. This harrowing realization was a wake-up call. I recognized that my health and safety, as well as that of my children, were at risk. It was in this moment of clarity that I knew I needed to seek help and make a change. This realization marked the beginning of my healing journey, leading me to seek medical support and holistic healing amid a whirlwind of symptoms and a diagnosis of complex post-traumatic stress disorder (PTSD).

Seeking Help

Despite extensive medical testing, a definitive cause for my distress remained elusive. A thorough psychological evaluation revealed stress-related physical symptoms and led to the diagnosis of PTSD. Understanding the root of my struggles was a crucial step in my path to healing.

The Revelation

Through this challenging period, I discovered that true well-being, peace, and joy are found within ourselves. This insight triggered a transformative shift towards self-love and alignment with my true self. Guided by the remarkable Deborah Clements, LMHC, and using techniques such as EMDR and EFT Tapping, I found strength and purpose amidst adversity.

Transformation and Healing

Emerging from this period of adversity, I discovered a renewed sense of self-love, inner peace, and resilience. The challenges and mental strain I faced, though initially unrecognized as postpartum depression (PPD), combined with emotional overwhelm and PTSD, became catalysts for my personal transformation and tools for helping others. My journey has ignited a deep passion for empowering mothers, assisting them in navigating their paths to optimal health and fulfillment in their motherhood journey.

Mission and Passion

My dedication to empowering mothers through holistic practices is unwavering. I believe that every mother deserves to experience the profound benefits of holistic health, from increased energy and mental clarity to emotional resilience and physical vitality. Through Inner Tranquility and our signature program, BlissfulBalance: The Ultimate

Wellness Package for Moms, I am committed to providing the guidance, support, and resources necessary for mothers to thrive.

Section 1: Understanding Maternal Wellness

Defining Holistic Maternal Health

Holistic maternal health encompasses the physical, emotional, and nutritional aspects of a mother's well-being. It is about nurturing the whole self and addressing the interconnectedness of mind, body, and spirit. A holistic approach considers not only the physiological changes during pregnancy and postpartum but also the emotional and mental well-being of the mother.

In my journey, I discovered that true wellness stems from addressing the root causes of our challenges, rather than just managing symptoms. By embracing holistic practices, we can achieve a balanced and harmonious state of health, enhancing our ability to thrive as mothers.

Unique Challenges

Motherhood is a journey filled with unique challenges at every stage, from preconception through postpartum. During preconception, the focus is on preparing the body for pregnancy, ensuring optimal nutrition, and managing stress. Pregnancy brings its own set of challenges, including hormonal changes, physical discomfort, and emotional fluctuations.

Postpartum, mothers face the demands of recovery, breastfeeding, and adapting to the new dynamics of motherhood. Each stage requires tailored support and guidance to navigate the complexities and promote overall well-being.

Section 2: The Holistic Approach to Motherhood

Holistic Healing Practices

Holistic healing practices play a vital role in supporting mothers' well-being. Mindset reprogramming, emotional wellness techniques, and stress management are essential components of this approach. Techniques such as mindfulness meditation, hypnotherapy, rapid transformational therapy (RTT®), emotional freedom technique (EFT Tapping), and eye movement desensitization and reprocessing (EMDR) have been instrumental in my healing journey.

These practices help mothers release negative emotions, overcome self-doubt, and cultivate a positive mindset. By addressing the emotional aspects of motherhood, we can create a foundation of inner peace and resilience.

Discovering Holistic Healing Practices

As a maternal health practitioner, my approach is rooted in holistic healing practices that address the unique needs of mothers at various stages of motherhood. While the specific modalities I use are essential, what truly matters is how these practices can transform your experience and enhance your well-being.

Prenatal and Postnatal Self-Care Routine

1. Prenatal Morning Mindfulness (5–10 minutes)

- **Purpose:** Start your day grounded and relaxed.

- **How-To:** Find a comfortable seated position and practice gentle breathing exercises or guided prenatal meditation. Focus on your breath and visualize a calm, nurturing environment for both you and your baby.

2. Balanced Prenatal/Postnatal Breakfast

- **Purpose:** Support your body's increased nutritional needs with organic food.

- **How-To:** Choose a breakfast rich in protein, healthy fats, and whole grains. For example, have a smoothie with spinach, berries, a scoop of plant-based protein powder, and chia seeds, or oatmeal topped with nuts and fruit.

3. Gentle Exercise Routine (10–15 minutes)

- **Purpose:** Maintain physical health and prepare for labor/ recovery.

- **How-To:** Engage in safe prenatal or postnatal exercises like gentle yoga stretches, pelvic floor exercises, or walking. Use online videos or apps designed for expectant and new mothers to ensure exercises are appropriate for your stage.

4. Hydration and Nutrient-Rich Snacks

- **Purpose:** Keep hydrated and maintain energy levels.

- **How-To:** Drink at least 8 glasses of water daily. Keep healthy snacks like sliced vegetables, fresh fruit, or nuts available to ensure you're getting the nutrients you and your baby need throughout the day.

5. Relaxation Time (10–15 minutes)

- **Purpose:** Reduce stress and promote mental well-being.

- **How-To:** Dedicate time to relaxation activities such as reading, gentle stretching, or listening to calming music. For postnatal moms, consider using this time for bonding with your baby through skin-to-skin contact or gentle baby massage.

6. Evening Wind-Down Ritual

- **Purpose:** Prepare for restful sleep and relaxation.

- **How-To:** Develop a calming bedtime routine that may include a warm bath with soothing essential oils, a cup of caffeine-free herbal tea, or light stretching. Create a quiet, dim environment to help your body wind down.

7. Weekly Self-Care Check-In

- **Purpose:** Address deeper needs and maintain overall well-being.

- **How-To:** Set aside time each week for a more focused self-care activity. This might include a prenatal massage, postnatal bodywork, or a relaxing bath. For prenatal care, consider creating a birth plan or attending a childbirth education class. For postnatal care, arrange for a support network check-in or engage in a postpartum exercise group.

Additional Tip: Incorporate mindfulness and breathing exercises throughout the day, particularly during moments of stress or when preparing for labor. This practice can help you stay centered and manage anxiety effectively.

These tailored strategies can help you maintain balance, support your physical and emotional health, and prepare for the joys and challenges of both pregnancy and the postpartum period.

What Being a Maternal Health Practitioner Means for You

Comprehensive Support: My role is to provide comprehensive support that encompasses physical, emotional, and mental well-being. This holistic approach ensures that you receive care tailored to every aspect of your health, helping you navigate the challenges of motherhood with greater ease and confidence.

Personalized Nutrition: Through personalized nutrition plans, I guide you in nourishing your body with the essential nutrients needed for energy, vitality, and overall wellness. These plans are designed to support you through pregnancy, postpartum recovery, and beyond, ensuring you and your baby receive optimal nourishment.

Mindset Coaching and Deep Healing: Motherhood can bring about significant emotional and psychological changes. My mindset coaching, combined with deep healing work using RTT®, helps you cultivate a positive and resilient mindset. This empowers you to manage stress, embrace self-care, and find joy in your daily life.

Rejuvenating Self-Care Practices: Self-care is vital for maintaining balance and well-being. I introduce rejuvenating self-care practices that fit seamlessly into your routine, promoting relaxation, reducing stress, and enhancing your overall quality of life.

The Benefits for You

Enhanced Well-Being: By integrating holistic practices into your life, you will experience enhanced physical and emotional well-being. This comprehensive care helps you feel more energized, balanced, and prepared to handle the demands of motherhood.

Empowerment and Confidence: With personalized guidance and support, you will feel empowered and confident in your journey. The tools and strategies you learn will help you make informed decisions about your health and your family's well-being.

Client Experience:

Embracing Motherhood with Confidence:

Sarah, a new mother, struggled with severe anxiety postpartum. Together, we uncovered the root cause of her anxiety and worked on reframing her mindset. As she progressed, she experienced a profound transformation. Her newfound confidence and emotional stability allowed her to embrace motherhood fully, enjoying the precious moments with her baby that anxiety once overshadowed.

Empowering Childbirth Experience:

Jessica, an expectant mother, was overwhelmed with uncertainty and worry about childbirth. Through our sessions and listening to the recording "Ease Into Pregnancy," she learned to visualize a calm and positive birth experience. This practice not only eased her fears but also contributed to a smoother and more empowering birthing process.

Rediscovering Joy and Vitality:

Emily, a mother of two, struggled with low energy, brain fog, and mood swings. Her daily life felt like a constant battle. We worked together to create a tailored nutrition plan, integrate mindfulness practices, and establish regular coaching sessions. Over time, she began to notice significant changes. She regained her energy, her mind became clearer, and her mood stabilized. She rediscovered joy in her daily life, feeling more present and connected with her children.

Nourishing with Nutrient-Dense Superfoods

Organic, premium, nutrient-dense superfoods are essential for holistic maternal health, providing vital vitamins, minerals, and antioxidants during pregnancy and postpartum. Products like Power Shake Nourishing Greens, Super Aminos, and Apothe-Cherry provide concentrated nutrients that boost vitality, support hormonal balance, and enhance overall well-being. Incorporating these superfoods into your daily routine addresses increased nutritional demands and promotes better health throughout pregnancy and the postpartum period.

Recommended Essentials for Maternal Wellness

First Trimester:

- **Power Shake Nourishing Greens:** Provides essential organic folate, beta carotene, and omega-3 fatty acids for fetal development and maternal health.

- **Super Aminos:** Supports skin elasticity, cell synthesis, and muscle tone, aiding post-birth recovery.

- **Biome Medic:** Maintains a healthy gut microbiome, reduces constipation, and eliminates glyphosate, benefiting both mother and baby.

- **Barley Juice:** Rich in organic micronutrients, folate, chlorophyll, and electrolytes, it supports healthy pH levels and cellular cleansing. Acts as a natural galactagogue to enhance breast milk production.

- **Cocoa Mint Spirulina:** Offers comprehensive nutrition, including organic B vitamins, iron, and omega fatty acids. Supports brain development, energy levels, and overall health.

- **Carrot Juice Plus:** Rich in organic carotenoids and antioxidants, it supports immune function and fetal development.

- **Zinc-Ade:** Enhances immune function and skin health.

- **Cracked Cell Chlorella:** Detoxifies heavy metals and supports cellular protection.

- **C from Nature:** Provides essential organic vitamin C, minerals, and antioxidants for overall health.

Optional Support for the First & Second Trimester:

- **Beet Juice:** Supports iron levels and energy.

- **Super Meal:** Provides comprehensive organic premium nutrition.

- **Aloe Digest:** Reduces gas, constipation, and UTI infections.

- **BIO Regen Caps:** Maintains mucosal lining health and elasticity.

- **Coconut Oil:** Helps prevent stretch marks and hemorrhoids, and increases skin elasticity.

- **Ginger:** Aids circulation, reduces nausea, and supports digestion.

Second & Third Trimester Addition's:

- **Dark Berry Protein:** Boosts energy and supports overall health with its blend of organic greens and vegetables.

- **Renew Hair, Skin & Nails:** Enhances collagen production, strengthens hair, nails, and skin, and supports stress relief.

- **Rice Bran Solubles:** Balances hormones and provides essential organic premium nutrients.

- **Bio Fruit:** Supports organic vitamin C intake and UTI prevention.

- **Coco Hydrate:** Contains organic premium electrolytes and antioxidants for joint support, hydration, and inflammation reduction.

- **Revive It All:** Enhances brain function, energy, and mental clarity.

- **MVP Family:** Adds extra organic vegan protein and organic whole food vitamin D.

Before Bed:

- **Apothe-Cherry:** Supports sleep and reduces inflammation with its organic, antioxidant-rich formula.

- **Ionic Elements:** Supplies essential organic minerals for vitality.

For Nursing Mothers:

- **ULT + Collagen Support:** It boosts energy and supports overall health with its organic premium greens and vegetable blend while promoting radiant skin, healthy hair growth, and joint health through enhanced collagen support.

- **Zinc-Ade:** Enhances immune support with essential organic vitamins and minerals.

- **Barley Green Juice:** Supports pH levels and natural milk production.

- **Ionic Elements:** Provides trace organic minerals for healthy hair, skin, and nails.

- **Carrot Juice Plus:** Improves organic vitamin A and beta-carotene levels in breast milk.

- **Rice Bran Solubles:** Supports hormone balance.

- **Revive It All:** Improves cognitive function and energy.

- **Coco Hydrate:** Provides hydration and anti-inflammatory benefits.

- **C from Nature:** Reinforces immune function and supports natural milk production.

- **Cocoa Mint Spirulina:** Prevents anemia, boosts immunity, and enhances the natural quality of breast milk.

These organic, premium, nutrient-dense superfoods offer comprehensive nutrition, eliminating the need for additional prenatal vitamins and ensuring both maternal and fetal health are supported throughout pregnancy and nursing.

Section 3: Practical Guidance for Mothers

Prenatal and Postpartum Nutrition

Proper nutrition is essential for both expectant and new mothers, supporting the baby's growth and the mother's recovery. A balanced diet rich in organic whole foods, lean proteins, healthy fats, and a variety of fruits and vegetables plays a key role in enhancing energy, stabilizing mood, and promoting overall health.

To support you on your wellness journey, I offer two transformative programs designed to meet you where you are and a free 5-Day Challenge:

- **Revive & Energize Postpartum: A 12-Week Reboot for Nurses**

  This 12-week journey offers a refreshing start for postpartum nurses ready to reclaim their energy, clarity, and resilience. Together, we'll take simple, foundational steps to help you feel more balanced and connected, using gentle guidance and practical self-care strategies. This program is all about helping you reconnect with yourself so you can actively enjoy motherhood while meeting the demands of your career with renewed strength.

- **BlissfulBalance: The Ultimate Wellness Package for Moms**

  For those ready to go deeper, this exclusive, year-long program allows you to work with me one-on-one to transform your health and well-being. As a health coach specializing in helping postpartum nurses overcome exhaustion, overwhelm, and brain fog, I'll guide you in boosting your energy, shedding postpartum weight, and actively enjoying motherhood.

With tailored nutrition plans, mindset coaching, and effective self-care strategies, you'll gain the tools to restore your energy, stabilize your mood, and create a more balanced and joyful motherhood experience. Plus, you'll enjoy an included virtual retreat and many other exciting bonuses designed to keep you supported and inspired throughout the year.

- **Free 5-Day Postpartum Refresh Challenge**

  If you're ready to take the first step toward feeling more energized and balanced, join my **Free 5-Day Postpartum Refresh Challenge** this December. It's an easy way to start incorporating some of the strategies I use to support postpartum health. For updates and details, join the **Postpartum Holistic Health and Recovery Facebook Group**, where the challenge dates will be announced soon.

  Join me for this transformative journey and feel your best as you embrace the joys of motherhood!

Supporting Mothers Through Every Stage

Preconception

Preconception is a crucial period to prepare your body for a healthy pregnancy. Optimal nutrition, stress management, and overall wellness are essential. Incorporating organic, premium, nutrient-dense superfoods, practicing mindfulness, and adopting a balanced lifestyle are key to supporting your journey into motherhood.

The Ultimate Lifestyle Transformation (ULT) program provides a comprehensive approach to preparing your body for conception. Key benefits include:

- **Organic Premium Nutrient-Dense Support for Optimal Health:** Ensures you receive essential nutrients crucial for fertility and preconception health, enhancing your chances of successful conception.

- **Balanced Energy:** Regulates energy levels, helping you stay vibrant and manage daily demands effectively.

- **Hormonal Balance:** Supports hormone regulation, beneficial for those with imbalances affecting fertility.

- **Detoxification:** Aids in eliminating toxins that could impact fertility, preparing your body for a healthy pregnancy.

- **Enhanced Immune Function:** Boosts your immune system to defend against illnesses that could affect pregnancy.

- **Optimized Digestion:** Promotes good gut health for efficient nutrient absorption, supporting reproductive health.

- **Mental Clarity and Emotional Well-Being:** Helps manage stress and maintain a positive mindset during the preconception period.

- **Overall Wellness:** Supports holistic well-being, laying a strong foundation for a healthy pregnancy and overall health.

Starting the ULT program for 90 days or more helps prepare both your body and mind for conception and pregnancy, ensuring a robust start for both you and your baby.

Pregnancy

Adopting holistic strategies during pregnancy can significantly enhance your experience. Prioritize prenatal nutrition by focusing on a diet rich in whole foods and superfoods. Incorporate practices such as hypnotherapy and mindfulness to manage stress and prepare for childbirth effectively.

The BlissfulBalance package offers comprehensive support throughout your motherhood journey. This holistic approach not only improves prenatal nutrition but also supports mental wellness with specialized guidance and resources tailored to your needs during pregnancy and postpartum. By blending personalized nutrition plans with mindset coaching and rejuvenating self-care practices, the BlissfulBalance package helps you navigate the emotional and physical changes of motherhood with greater ease and grace, ensuring a harmonious and fulfilling experience.

Postpartum

The postpartum period requires special care and attention. Focus on recovery, nutrition, and emotional well-being. Incorporate superfoods to support healing, your body needs support to recover and thrive. Focus on nutrient-dense superfoods to replenish your body's stores, support breastfeeding, and promote healing and sustained energy. Safe superfood regimens such as ULT + Collagen can further support maternal health during this critical period.

Engage in practices like RTT® and health coaching to address any challenges you may face. Incorporate emotional wellness techniques like EFT Tapping and regular mindfulness practices to navigate the new dynamics of motherhood with resilience and grace.

Managing Stress and Energy

Balancing motherhood with personal well-being requires effective stress management and energy-boosting strategies. Mindfulness practices, such as deep breathing exercises and meditation, can help reduce stress and promote relaxation. Regular physical activity, adequate sleep, and self-care routines are also vital for maintaining energy levels and overall well-being.

In my experience, creating a structured daily routine that includes time for self-care, mindfulness, and nourishing meals can make a significant difference in managing stress and maintaining energy throughout the day.

Section 4: Supporting Mothers Through Challenges

Addressing Hormonal Balance

Hormonal changes during and after pregnancy can significantly impact a mother's well-being. Holistic approaches to managing hormonal balance include proper nutrition, stress reduction, and specific superfoods known for their hormone-supporting properties. Organic foods rich in omega-3 fatty acids, such as flaxseeds and chia seeds, can help regulate hormones and reduce inflammation.

Additionally, adaptogenic herbs like organic ashwagandha and maca can support adrenal health and promote hormonal balance. Integrating these natural remedies into your diet can help alleviate symptoms of hormonal imbalance and support overall health.

Enhancing Digestive Health

Digestive health is crucial for overall well-being, especially during pregnancy and postpartum. The gut plays a vital role in nutrient absorption, immune function, and mental health. A diet rich in fiber, probiotics, and prebiotics can support digestive health and promote a balanced gut microbiome.

Organic Premium Superfood Supplements like Biome Medic and Rice Bran Solubles can help enhance gut health and reduce inflammation. By prioritizing digestive health, mothers can improve nutrient absorption, boost energy levels, and support overall wellness.

Section 5: Building a Supportive Community

Creating Connections

Community support is essential for maternal health. Connecting with other mothers who share similar experiences can provide a sense of belonging and understanding. Sharing stories, challenges, and triumphs can create a supportive network that fosters emotional well-being.

Engaging in community activities, such as wellness workshops and support groups, can help mothers feel empowered and connected. Online platforms and social media groups also offer valuable opportunities for creating meaningful connections and sharing resources.

Engagement and Empowerment

The **Postpartum Holistic Health and Recovery** group, along with the Wellness Warriors virtual gathering and the Million Mom Movement, is dedicated to empowering mothers through education, engagement, and shared experiences. Our supportive network is designed to create a positive environment where you can connect with others who understand your journey.

We offer access to a wealth of educational resources, including webinars, articles, and books, to help you make informed decisions about your health and well-being. By participating in wellness challenges, such as mindful eating or fitness goals, you can foster a sense of accomplishment and motivation, further enhancing your personal growth and health journey.

Our community gatherings and initiatives are designed to celebrate successes and share experiences, creating a space where mothers uplift and support one another. The **Postpartum Holistic Health and Recovery** group provides a platform for this connection, while the Wellness Warriors virtual gatherings every Wednesday offer real-time interaction and community engagement. Additionally, the Million Mom

Movement connects you with a broader initiative focused on the importance of nutrition and wellness.

Together, these efforts build a vibrant and empowering community where each member contributes to a nurturing and supportive environment. By engaging with these communities, you not only find encouragement but also become part of a collective effort to achieve optimal health, well-being, and joy in your motherhood journey.

Engaging with Our Community

Wellness Community Gatherings

We host a Wellness Community Gathering every Wednesday, where we come together to share experiences, support each other, and explore holistic wellness practices. This gathering is a space for connection, learning, and mutual encouragement. It is a place where you can find inspiration, share your journey, and gain insights from others who are on a similar path.

Referral Program: Share the Bliss, Reap the Rewards

I deeply value the power of community and the collective support of those who share our mission. That's why I'm excited to introduce my Referral Program, designed to celebrate and reward you for spreading the word about **BlissfulBalance: The Ultimate Wellness Package for Moms**.

Here's How It Works:

1. **Refer Three Friends:** Spread the joy of BlissfulBalance by referring three individuals who sign up for the full program.

2. **Choose Your Reward:**

   - **$250 Off Any Transformational Package:** Enjoy a

significant discount on any of our transformational packages (not including superfood products).

- **Customizable Transformational Recording:** Receive a personalized recording valued at $250 to support your ongoing journey to wellness.

It's our way of saying thank you for helping others embark on their path to well-being. Your referrals not only contribute to our growing community but also help more mothers discover the transformative benefits of the BlissfulBalance package.

Start sharing today and enjoy the rewards of making a difference!

Testimonials and Success Stories

Real-life testimonials showcase the powerful impact of our programs and build trust within our community.

Vanessa's Transformation:

Vanessa, a business owner and mother of three, faced a challenging diagnosis of Multiple Sclerosis (MS), Rheumatoid Arthritis (RA), Scleroderma, and high blood pressure. Despite her doctors' recommendations for lifelong medication, Vanessa sought alternative solutions.

Through the ULT 90-Day Program, Vanessa experienced a remarkable recovery within 45 days, reversing her diagnoses and symptoms. Despite this incredible progress, Vanessa felt something was still missing in her life. She decided to explore hypnotherapy, which led to a profound shift in her outlook and well-being. The immediate results were life-changing; she overcame negative thoughts, and fears of success, and felt a renewed sense of fulfillment.

Vanessa now shares her journey to inspire others, demonstrating the transformative potential of holistic approaches and self-advocacy.

Promotions and Special Offers

To further support your journey, we have special promotions for my 90-day ULT Superfood Program. When you purchase the nutritional program, you will receive a free on-the-go rechargeable blender with your first ULT kit purchase, plus a 25% gift code to use on your first and subsequent purchases. This offer enhances the convenience of incorporating superfoods into your daily routine and provides additional value to your investment in holistic health.

Section 6: Partnering with Holistic Practitioners

The Role of Holistic Maternal Health Practitioners

As a holistic maternal health practitioner, I provide essential support through personalized nutrition plans, mindset coaching, and overall wellness strategies tailored to each mother's unique needs. By integrating these approaches, I help mothers navigate the complexities of pregnancy and postpartum with confidence and resilience. Real-life testimonials illustrate the transformative impact of holistic care, showcasing how personalized support can significantly enhance maternal well-being.

Collaboration with Birth Workers and Doulas

Collaboration with birth workers and doulas enhances the care provided during pregnancy, childbirth, and the postpartum period. While birth workers and doulas focus on emotional and physical support, I concentrate on holistic health practices, including nutrition and emotional well-being. This collaborative approach ensures mothers receive comprehensive care that addresses their needs from multiple angles, promoting a well-rounded and fulfilling experience throughout their journey.

Looking Forward

My goal is to expand services, launch new products, and further contribute to maternal wellness. I'm committed to empowering mothers through holistic practices and nutrient-dense nourishment.

I'm excited to enhance the Revive & Energize Postpartum: A 12-Week Reboot and Blissful Balance program, adding new features and resources to better support your journey. These programs are integral to my mission of providing personalized care and holistic support, helping you achieve optimal health and joy in motherhood.

Holistic maternal health encompasses physical, emotional, and nutritional well-being. By integrating holistic practices, superfoods, and community support, mothers can attain radiant health from preconception to postpartum.

Though the journey to empowerment has its challenges, with the right tools and support, every mother can thrive. Prioritize your well-being and embrace holistic practices and superfoods to build a healthy and fulfilling motherhood. Remember, you're not alone—together, we can create a supportive community that uplifts each other.

A Gift To YOU, as a thank you!

Ultimately LifeStyle Transformation: $100 OFF

Gift Code:
https://ishoppurium.com/Ultlifestyle?giftcard=5683LoveLife

Appendix

Resources and Recommendations

For further exploration of holistic maternal health and wellness, here are additional resources, recommended readings, and links:

BOOKS & BLOGS

- Decoding Baby Blues & Postpartum Struggles
- https://blog.puriumcorp.com/2020/05/14/nutrition-for-new-mothers/
- https://cdn.ishoppurium.store/The-Toxin-that-Came-to-Dinner.pdf

WEBSITES & VIRTUAL COMMUNITIES FOR MOTHERS

- innertranquility.life
- https://www.facebook.com/share/g/19qGhpi9yJ/

RECOMMENDED SUPERFOOD PRODUCTS & SUPPLEMENT

- ULT + Collagen & Blissful Balance: The Ultimate Wellness Package for Moms

CONTACTS

- npatterson@innertranquility.life
- P: 727-244-7519
- https://calendly.com/innertranquility/breakthroughsession
- https://calendly.com/innertranquility/wellnesscheckin

SOCIAL MEDIA

- https://www.facebook.com/innertranquility.life?mibextid=LQQJ4d
- https://www.instagram.com/innertranquility.life?igsh=NHJ3emh1cnpsNmd4&utm_source=qr

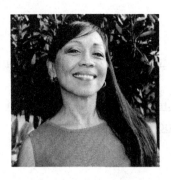

Carol Cretella

Founder of Carol Cretella

https://www.linkedin.com/in/carol-cretella-a67504233
https://www.facebook.com/carol.cretella.16/
https://www.instagram.com/carol.cretella/
https://carolcretella.com/

Carol Cretella is a 69 year-old yoga/pilates instructor and Feminine Embodiment Coach who still does headstands, full splits and other fun poses.

Carol had a successful career in the New York Fashion Industry but the long hours and high stress resulted chronic health issues for her. She left that career to enter a Yoga Teacher Training in 2005 and never looked back.

As a feminine embodiment coach, Carol works with women who want to look and feel healthy, energetic, youthful, and radiant but struggle with weight gain, physical pain, and a lack of consistent follow through to create lasting change in their lives. Carol teaches women to take control of their lives by accessing their innate feminine wisdom and by listening and trusting their own inner guidance so they can look and feel their radiant best and attract what they want in life.

To learn more about Carol's services, coaching, and retreats, visit carolcretella.com and her YouTube channel (Carol Cretella).

INNER WEALTH:
The Key to Fulfillment and Happiness

By Carol Cretella

I became a Health and Wellness Coach because I saw a common scenario among women. Many women pursue their dreams of an ideal life by working longer and harder at their jobs or as entrepreneurs in addition to raising their families, volunteering for community service, and/or caring for aging parents. It's common to see women overwhelmed, juggling so much and putting their own needs aside because our culture tells us that we must be Superwomen. It's stressful and exhausting and comes at the cost of body, mind, and spirit.

Does this resonate with you? Are you going through the motions of running on a never-ending treadmill of activity, yet feeling that something is missing in life?

That was my story. I wanted to achieve my vision of prosperity, fulfillment, and happiness. I still want that for me and I want that for you. We can achieve that—with FULL health and inner peace.

MY JOURNEY

Ever since I was a child growing up in Hawaii, I wanted to be a fashion designer. I followed that dream all the way to NYC, attended college there, and stayed to forge a career.

To my twenty-one-year-old self, the fashion industry was intoxicating. On one hand, intoxicating means enticing and exhilarating. On the other hand, it means impairment of judgment and senses. I was young and addicted.

I worked my way up through a series of jobs that were fast-paced, challenging...grueling. The deadlines were demanding, but I was determined to do what it took to become a success. I worked my way up until I landed a job as head designer. My first line was a huge success. At the rate I was going, marriage and motherhood were not in the picture.

But then Andrew came along. He convinced me that there was more to life than just my career. We fell in love, got married, and four years later, had a beautiful baby boy.

After I had my baby, I wanted to keep it all: career, motherhood, AND a lovely home in the suburbs. I had just landed an exciting new job as head designer of a start-up company, and I was determined to make it a success.

This was my weekday routine: 5 hours of sleep, get up at 5 a.m., drop off my baby at daycare, and take the train to Manhattan; work all day at my fast-paced, demanding job with constantly changing deadlines; after work, commute back to Long Island, race to pick up my son by 6:30 p.m., and then go home to my other job as Mom. Meals were pizza, pasta, or take-out.

Professionally, I got what I wanted. The company became successful and grew rapidly. Things were going great, but in the back of my mind, the FEAR of reversal of fortune reared its ugly head. There's a saying in the fashion industry: "A designer is only as good as his or her last line." So I felt the pressure to work longer, harder, faster.

But sadly, in my heart, I began to yearn for a simpler life.

I eventually developed a chronic case of asthma. I kept inhalers around everywhere. My weight crept up until I was about twenty pounds overweight. The neck and shoulder pain I had from a car accident years ago never healed. It just did not occur to me that my health issues were caused by constant stress.

One night, my asthma was worse than usual, but I shrugged it off. My husband was away on a business trip, and I was home alone with a cranky, crying baby. Finally, I put my son to bed, did some chores, and went to bed past midnight. When I lay down, I felt like there were a ton of bricks on my chest. I could not breathe while lying down. I could only breathe when sitting up. The inhalers didn't help. My mind was fuzzy at this point, and I thought, "I can't go to the emergency room, who will take care of my baby?" So I spent the rest of the night awake, sitting up and pushing out every breath. I believe that if I had not willed myself to push out every breath all night long, I would have died.

When the sun rose in the morning, I was never so happy to see a sunrise. I took my baby to daycare and took myself to the emergency room.

That was my wake-up call. After that experience, I finally acknowledged to myself the dreaded "B" word: BURN-OUT! I had been listening to my head and not the inner whisperings of my heart and soul. The consequence of ignoring the subconscious communication of our inner selves is that the soul sends increasingly "louder" messages like irritability, fatigue, depression, poor health, and eventually, chronic disease.

All of the symptoms I listed amount to a cry of the soul for attention. In my case, it culminated that one fateful night when I almost died of an asthma attack. That was the turning point in my life. I knew I had to make some major changes.

With my husband's help, I committed to reimagining my health and my life. But it had taken a very long time for me and my body to break down. It was going to take not just time but research, trial and error, and discipline to rebuild the health of my body, mind, and spirit.

I joined a gym and started working out regularly. Through commitment and consistency, exercise became a "non-negotiable" part of my life. I took it another step further and enrolled in a tennis class. It was fun and social, and it was great exercise. I became hooked on an activity that is healthy in many aspects!

However, although my physical health improved, the nature of the industry I worked in was not going to change. What I really needed to do was change careers. But what else could I do? I had no idea.

One day at work, I met Dana, a textile saleswoman. I admired Dana's radiant, healthy presence and fit physique. She exuded calm and groundedness. She mentioned that she taught yoga on the weekends and had a plan to open up her own yoga studio. I was intrigued and captivated by her vision. I remembered back to when I practiced yoga regularly in college. My yoga practice made my body feel toned, strong, and flexible. The yoga breathing practices and meditation allowed me to feel calm and present.

The gears in my head started turning. I asked myself, "Me—a yoga instructor?" I have to admit, the thought of giving up a lucrative career to become a yoga instructor seemed ludicrous, but my heart soared at the thought of helping others to improve their health. I started attending yoga classes again, and it was like going back home to a place that had been so nurturing before. When the time arrived to make a change, I was ready and never looked back. I enrolled in yoga teacher training and became a certified yoga instructor.

My yoga career, among other holistic disciplines that I have pursued, allowed me to create the Inner Wealth that provides me with satisfaction, fulfillment, and happiness in my life.

WHAT IS INNER WEALTH?

As I see it, true wealth is Inner Wealth, which cannot be bought. I define Inner Wealth as having abundant inner resources of radiant health, inner peace, love, positivity, and gratitude so we can meet life's challenges and create joy and fulfillment. Inner Wealth also includes sharing the wealth by playing a part in making the world a more peaceful, and empowered place—starting with ourselves, then spreading the love to our families, communities, and the world.

Where do we find these resources? The answer is literally within—Inner Wealth is inside of us, waiting to be discovered, cultivated, and shared with others.

FIVE COMPONENTS OF INNER WEALTH

I've identified five components of Inner Wealth:

1) Health of Mind, Body, and Spirit

Optimum health is the harmonious balance between mind, body, and spirit. Each element is critical to our overall health. When each element is nurtured, they cultivate a sense of fulfillment that money cannot buy.

Mind

Think of your mind as your inner playground. The ability to think clearly can shape everything in our lives, from making sound decisions more easily, to coping with stress effectively. Practices such as mindfulness, meditation, and continuous learning can help sharpen our minds and strengthen emotional fortitude. By nurturing our minds, we create a positive internal dialogue that fuels our dreams and goals and enhances self-worth.

Body

Physical health is super important because it impacts our mood and energy levels. Our bodies are our "earth suits" in which we experience the world. Caring for them through healthy eating, regular exercise, and adequate rest enables us to fully participate in life. A strong and healthy body not only increases energy but also contributes to mental clarity and emotional stability. When we prioritize our physical well-being, we lay a solid foundation for cultivating Inner Wealth.

Spirit

This aspect of Inner Wealth has to do with our values, our place in the world, beliefs, and sense of purpose. We can nurture our spiritual health in many ways, such as connecting with nature, engaging in community service, or exploring spiritual practices. This exploration fosters a deeper connection and understanding of ourselves and our place in the world. When our spirit is nurtured, we experience a sense of connection to something greater than ourselves, enhancing feelings of gratitude and contentment.

2) PEACE

Imagine waking up each day with a sense of calm and balance. How can we navigate through life's ups and downs without feeling overwhelmed? You can find your inner peace through practices like meditation, spending time in nature, or just taking a moment to breathe deeply. It's about creating a sanctuary within ourselves, where we can retreat anytime life gets a bit hectic.

3) LOVE

Love and compassion for ourselves and others create Inner Wealth. Self-love is especially powerful in that it fosters self-acceptance, enabling us to embrace our imperfections and acknowledge our self-worth. When we love ourselves, we are better able to extend that love to others, building strong and supportive relationships. Acts of kindness, gratitude, and simply being present for someone can create a ripple effect of positivity. Love makes our lives more meaningful and helps us feel supported, which is so important for our overall happiness!

4) POSITIVITY

Positivity is far more than having a cheerful, optimistic outlook. It is an essential component of Inner Wealth that can shape our experiences and our interactions with the world. A positive mindset can really transform how we see the world. It helps us to face challenges head-on and inspires us to keep moving forward. You can boost your positivity by journaling, practicing affirmations, and surrounding yourself with uplifting people.

5) GRATITUDE

Gratitude is like a little spark that lights up your day. We can practice creating a feeling of abundance by appreciating the good things in our lives, no matter how big or small. Practicing gratitude immediately shifts our focus from lack to what we already have—like finding a treasure in our own backyard! Simple ways to experience the power of gratitude are jotting down three things you're grateful for each day, expressing thanks to others, and taking moments for mindfulness that can help us appreciate everyday joys.

YOGA—A MULTI-PURPOSE DISCIPLINE FOR CREATING INNER WEALTH

YOGA is one of the best practices for uniting mind, body, and spirit and cultivating peace, love, positivity, and gratitude!

With its mix of physical postures, breathing techniques, and meditation, yoga helps us to become more self-aware and present. Not only does it strengthen and relax our bodies, but it also calms our minds, which cuts down on stress and boosts emotional resilience. As we quiet our minds and slow down the busy pace of life, we can connect more deeply within ourselves and find a sense of peace and fulfillment. I encourage you to make yoga a regular part of your life. You may find that it enhances your overall well-being and helps to develop a greater appreciation for yourself and the world around you.

THE TAKEAWAY

It was a long journey from where I was to where I am today. The asthma is completely gone, it's a thing of my distant past. I easily maintain my ideal weight without fighting myself. The neck and shoulder pain is minimal because I exercise and practice yoga regularly. The Inner Wealth that I have cultivated, nurtured, and maintained over the years has served me well in pursuing my health and wellness career. I currently apply my knowledge and skills as a Yoga instructor, Art of Feminine Presence Teacher, Certified Transformational Life Coach, and Therapeutic Art instructor to the programs of Women's Wellness Retreats that I host throughout the year.

Inner Wealth is all about nurturing the health of our mind, body, and spirit while cultivating peace, love, positivity, and gratitude. By focusing on these elements, we can create a life filled with meaning, fulfillment, and joy. In a world that often emphasizes material wealth, it's vital to remember that true riches lie within us—waiting to be explored, nurtured, and shared with others. Embracing this journey allows us to enhance our own lives and positively impact those around us.

Let's prioritize Inner Wealth and create lives that are truly fulfilling and joyful!

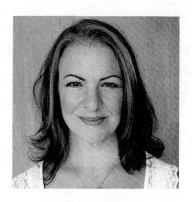

Sue Ellar

Eat Well Feel Great
Health, Vitality & Weight Loss Coach

https://uk.linkedin.com/in/sueellar
https://www.facebook.com/sueellar/
https://www.instagram.com/sue.ellar/
https://sueellar.com/
https://linktr.ee/sueellar

Sue Ellar is a Health Transformation Coach who helps women over 40 reclaim their vitality, energy, body confidence and ideal weight by embracing a healthier relationship with food.

After decades of battling weight gain and yo-yo dieting, Sue discovered the life-changing power of the natural human diet to dramatically transform her health, boost energy, and achieve lasting weight loss while reducing chronic symptoms. This profound transformation inspired her to leave her IT career to become a Master WILDFIT® coach.

With compassion, enthusiasm, and deep personal experience, Sue has guided nearly 200 clients to break free from emotional eating and achieve lasting results.

Sue's approach blends evolutionary nutrition with food psychology, making sustainable changes enjoyable. She now lives her dream lifestyle, working with clients all over the world, and is on a mission to spark a ripple effect of positive change by empowering the changemakers of the world with this method.

Breaking Free: From Dieting to Empowerment

By Sue Ellar

1. Introduction and History

Over the years, I've come to realise that the journey to better health isn't just about what we eat—it's about the mindset we bring to our relationship with food.

For much of my life, I battled with my weight, self-image, and the emotional rollercoaster that comes with yo-yo dieting. As a child, I may have had a bit of puppy fat, but in reality, I looked like any other kid. And yet, for decades, I became caught in a cycle of restrictive dieting and emotional eating, desperately trying to control my weight.

But the more I restricted myself, the more I craved the very foods I was trying to avoid. Dieting became a relentless battle between what I wanted to eat and what I thought I should eat, and I lost that battle repeatedly.

The diets I tried were endless—Slimming World, low-fat regimes, calorie counting—but none of them brought the lasting results I longed for. Instead, they made eating a miserable experience, stripping away the joy and replacing it with guilt and shame. My self-worth became tied to the number on the scale, and each failed attempt only deepened my sense of failure. I was trapped in a vicious cycle, feeling both powerless and frustrated.

Looking back, I see that my relationship with food was deeply dysfunctional. I used food not just to satisfy hunger but to fill emotional voids, to soothe, and to reward myself. I believed that food needed to be indulgent, that it had to bring comfort and satisfaction, but I had no idea what it meant to use food as a tool for health. This cycle of deprivation and overindulgence continued into adulthood, exacerbated by the pressures of daily life and the demands of being a mother.

It wasn't until my forties that I realised the key to breaking free from this cycle was not just changing what I ate, but transforming how I thought about food. Dieting wasn't working because it was based on deprivation and punishment, not on nourishing my body or caring for myself. A shift in my mindset—sparked by new insights and approaches—began to change how I viewed food and health, laying the groundwork for the transformation that was to come.

But the real turning point came in 2020 when I found a new approach that was unlike anything I had tried before. This method wasn't about deprivation or counting calories; it focused on understanding the body's needs and nourishing it with natural, wholesome foods. For the first time, I began to truly listen to my body, recognising the different types of hunger and learning how to make choices that supported my health rather than undermining it.

The transformation was profound. I lost weight, but more importantly, I gained a new sense of freedom. I no longer felt trapped by the cycle of dieting and bingeing. Instead, I felt empowered to make choices that made me feel vibrant, healthy, and alive. For the first time, I understood the importance of having a "Big Why"—a reason so compelling that it motivated me to eat for health, not out of obligation or guilt.

This journey has been about so much more than weight loss. It's been about reclaiming my health, my energy, and my confidence. It's about the joy of waking up each morning with vitality, the pleasure of nourishing my body with foods that make me feel good, and the freedom that comes from breaking free from the chains of dieting. And now, I'm on a mission to share this journey with others, to empower them to take control of their health, and to show them that a better relationship with food is not just possible—it's within reach for everyone.

2. Early Challenges: A Life Shaped by Dieting and Emotional Eating

My struggle with food and body image began at an alarmingly young age. I was only nine years old when a boy at school made a cruel comment about my weight: "You're so fat that even if you didn't eat for a month, you'd still be fat," he sneered. That comment planted a seed of self-doubt that would grow and entangle itself in every aspect of my life for decades. Looking back at photos from that time, I realise I was just a normal kid with perhaps a bit of puppy fat. But those words—along with a particularly unflattering photo—became etched into my mind, and from that point on, I began to see myself as "the fat person."

As I moved into my teenage years, that identity solidified. I became painfully self-conscious about my body, especially my developing figure. I obsessed over my size, often trying to squeeze into jeans that were too small, leading to physical discomfort and pain. It wasn't just about how I looked; it was about how I felt in my own skin. I believed that if I could just lose a bit of weight, I'd be happy. But the more I tried, the more I seemed to fail.

Our family meals didn't make things any easier. Midweek dinners were often quick and easy options like burgers, sausages, or fish fingers—foods that weren't exactly conducive to a healthy lifestyle. Sundays, however, were different. My dad would prepare a glorious roast dinner with a spread of vegetables, but even then, there was always an expectation to clear your plate, leading to an uncomfortable sense of overfullness that I struggled to manage. This pattern of eating—alternating between indulgence and restriction—became ingrained, and I carried it into adulthood.

As I grew older, this dysfunctional relationship with food only intensified. I vividly remember how, after arguments with boyfriends or during moments of emotional turmoil, I would turn to food for comfort. Late-night trips to the chip shop for fish and chips became a regular coping mechanism. I wasn't just eating out of hunger; I was eating to fill an emotional void, to soothe the pain or frustration I felt. Food became both a source of comfort and distress, trapping me in a cycle of emotional eating that I couldn't seem to escape.

In my twenties and thirties, my social life was buzzing. Every week was filled with meals out, drinks with friends, and endless gatherings—all centred around food. I loved being out and about, but it made sticking to any diet nearly impossible. Food was more than just nourishment; it was part of every celebration and connection. Yet, each indulgence brought a wave of guilt, fueling a constant battle between enjoying life and trying to control my weight. My vibrant social life, while full of joy, only deepened my struggle with food and self-image.

This cycle of deprivation and overindulgence, of guilt and self-loathing, persisted for years. I became increasingly desperate, searching for a way to break free from the patterns that were holding me back. But the more I tried to control my eating, the more out of control I felt. And it was exhausting.

3. The Turning Point

By the time I reached my forties, I began to see that traditional dieting wasn't just making me miserable; it was actually working against me. The more I tried to restrict and control what I ate, the more my body seemed to rebel. I'd feel colder, more tired, and no slimmer for all the effort. It dawned on me that these so-called "diet foods" I was forcing down were actually doing more harm than good—they were unhealthy, unsatisfying, and left me feeling worse off.

Around that time, I started exploring different ideas, like low-GI diets and food combining. These approaches made more sense to me and got me thinking that maybe there was a better, more natural way to eat. It wasn't an overnight shift, but gradually, I realised that dieting was never going to be the answer. I had to stop following restrictive diets that were clearly not working and start focusing on nourishing my body in a way that felt right.

That was the moment I decided to ditch dieting for good. I stopped punishing myself with calorie counting and started searching for a more mindful, sustainable approach to food and health. I learned that long-term success wasn't about punishing myself or exercising willpower, but about changing the way I thought about food. This was a revelation. For the first time, I began to understand that my struggles weren't just about food; they were about the way I approached food and my relationship with it.

In 2020, I discovered a revolutionary approach to health that would forever change my relationship with food: WILDFIT®. Unlike the countless diets I had tried before, WILDFIT® wasn't about restriction or calorie counting. Instead, it was based on understanding the body's natural needs and nourishing it with the foods we are biologically designed to eat. The programme emphasises the importance of listening to your body, recognising different types of hunger, and making food choices that support overall health and well-being. WILDFIT® provided me with a framework that made sense on a fundamental level, transforming not just my body, but my mindset and approach to life itself.

The transformation was exhilarating. Within weeks of starting the WILDFIT® 90-day challenge, I noticed significant changes. My energy levels soared, my sleep quality improved, and the joint pain that had plagued me for years began to fade. I released 14 pounds of fat and dropped a dress size. My face, especially around the eyes, looked less puffy, and I felt more vibrant and alive than I had in years. These changes weren't just physical; they were emotional, too. I no longer felt trapped by the cycle of dieting and bingeing. Instead, I felt empowered to make choices that supported my health and well-being.

But the most profound change was in my relationship with food. I began to see food not as a source of guilt or as a battleground, but as a tool for nourishment and health. I learned to eat in a way that felt natural and sustainable. The constant craving for unhealthy foods diminished, and I found myself genuinely enjoying foods that I had once viewed as boring or unsatisfying. For the first time in my life, I felt in control of my eating habits, and it was liberating.

4. From Personal Journey to Empowering Clients

My transformation was profound. I reclaimed my health, my identity, and a newfound sense of freedom and control. This wasn't just about losing weight or improving my diet; it was about reclaiming my health and my identity. I knew that I couldn't keep this to myself—I needed to help others who were struggling as I had been.

When the opportunity to become a WILDFIT® coach came along, I jumped at the chance. It was a significant investment, both financially and emotionally, but I knew it was the right path for me. The results I had seen in my own life and in the lives of others were undeniable, and I felt a deep sense of purpose in helping others achieve the same transformation.

Over the next two years, I helped dozens of clients break free from the cycle of dieting, regain their health, and discover a new way of living. This journey not only transformed my clients' lives but also deepened my commitment to the work I was doing. At the time, I was still working at Cardiff University, juggling a demanding job with family life and my own health goals. But deep down, I knew that this was the right path. I had seen firsthand the life-changing results that WILDFIT® could deliver, not just for me but for others as well.

After completing my certification and starting part-time, I was initially nervous, but the miraculous transformations I witnessed quickly dispelled any doubts. People who had been trapped in cycles of dieting and self-loathing were suddenly discovering a new way of living, one that didn't require willpower or deprivation, but rather a deeper understanding and respect for their bodies.

One of my earliest clients, Donna, was a life coach herself but had been diagnosed with long COVID, type 2 diabetes, and fibromyalgia. These conditions had dramatically altered her life, leaving her exhausted and unable to enjoy the activities she once loved. Over the course of 90 days, we worked together to overhaul her diet and mindset. The results were astounding. She went from struggling to get out of bed to walking 18 miles and swimming 160 lengths. She lost three and a half stone and reversed her type 2 diabetes. Her story was just one of many that reaffirmed my belief in the power of WILDFIT® and my role as a coach.

—Justine had been living with chronic back pain for over 20 years, which severely affected her quality of life. After joining my programme, she experienced a dramatic transformation. She went from struggling to get out of bed each morning to moving with ease, eventually shedding over 12 kgs. Her chronic pain diminished significantly, and she regained a sense of energy and confidence she hadn't felt in decades. Justine's journey is a powerful testament to the impact of the right guidance and support in achieving lasting health improvements.

Now, having guided nearly 200 clients through the programme, including my own parents who overcame their type 2 diabetes, I see this work not just as a career but as a mission. Each success story is a reminder of why I do what I do. I'm excited to continue this journey, to help more people break free from the constraints of dieting and poor health, and to guide them towards a life of vitality and empowerment. This isn't just about changing lives—it's about changing the world, one healthy choice at a time.

5. Understanding ADHD and Food Relationships

As I continued on my journey towards better health, a new and profound realisation emerged—one that would add another layer of understanding to my lifelong struggle with food. It wasn't until late 2022 that I began to fully grasp the impact of undiagnosed ADHD and Autism (PDA) on my relationship with food. This realisation brought clarity to behaviours and patterns that I had wrestled with for years but had never fully understood.

Growing up, I was always a bit rebellious, especially when it came to being told what to eat. Diet programmes that imposed strict rules and limitations always backfired on me. I found myself resisting these restrictions, not because I didn't want to be healthier, but because the rigidity of these programmes clashed with something deep within me. It wasn't until I recognised the signs of ADHD that I began to understand why.

ADHD is often characterised by impulsivity, difficulty with focus, and a tendency to seek out instant gratification. For years, I struggled with impulsive eating, driven by intense cravings that seemed to come out of nowhere. Supermarket shopping was a particularly overwhelming experience. I would walk into the store with a vague idea of what I needed, only to be bombarded by endless options and conflicting thoughts—should I be saving money, cutting out junk food, or trying something new? Should I go down every aisle or just stick to the essentials? The sheer number of decisions was paralysing.

This constant bombardment of choices led to a phenomenon known as "decision fatigue," which made it even harder to make healthy choices. Often, I found myself reaching for foods that provided a quick dopamine hit—chocolate, crisps, or a glass of wine—because they offered immediate satisfaction in a world that often felt overwhelming. These cravings weren't just about hunger; they were about seeking relief from the constant noise and chaos in my mind.

Understanding that my ADHD was driving these behaviours was a game-changer. It allowed me to approach food and eating in a way that acknowledged my need for immediate rewards, without sacrificing my long-term health goals. I realised that in order to maintain a healthy diet, I needed to find foods and strategies that provided quick satisfaction but in a way that was aligned with my overall well-being.

This insight has profoundly influenced the way I now coach my health transformation clients. I emphasise the importance of finding personal, tactile benefits—like increased energy, better sleep, and reduced inflammation—that provide immediate rewards. For clients with ADHD, these tangible benefits are crucial because they offer the quick feedback that our brains crave. It's not just about eating because we should; it's about eating because we want to feel good in the moment and in the long run.

I also focus on practical strategies that make healthy eating more accessible and less overwhelming. For instance, I coach my clients on the importance of easy food prep—having ready-made, nutritious options that can be grabbed on the go. This reduces the decision-making burden and makes it easier to stick to healthy habits, especially on days when energy and focus are in short supply.

Another cornerstone of my coaching approach is fostering a positive and non-judgmental mindset. I encourage my clients to view their food choices not as successes or failures, but as learning experiences. When someone tells me they've "lost the plot" or "not stuck to it," I help them find the positive aspects of what they've done and celebrate the progress they've made. This approach is vital, especially for those with ADHD, because it shifts the focus from guilt and shame to empowerment and growth.

In many ways, my journey with ADHD has been one of self-discovery and acceptance. It has taught me that health isn't about rigid rules or perfection; it's about finding what works for you as an individual. By integrating these insights into my coaching, I'm able to help my clients not only achieve their health goals but also develop a healthier, more compassionate relationship with themselves. And for me, that's what true health is all about.

6. Building a Movement: Empowering Change on a Larger Scale

As my personal transformation took hold and I began to see the profound impact on my own life, I knew I couldn't keep this knowledge to myself. The changes I experienced were too powerful, too life-altering, to remain confined within the boundaries of my own experience. I felt a calling—a deep, undeniable urge to share what I had learned with as many people as possible. This was about more than just health; it was about creating a ripple effect that could transform lives on a much larger scale.

The decision to become a WILDFIT® coach was the first step in what has since become a much larger mission. I was no longer content with simply improving my own health; I wanted to help others experience the same freedom and empowerment that I had found. This wasn't just about weight loss or physical well-being—it was about reclaiming control over one's life and making conscious, intentional choices that aligned with personal values and long-term goals.

As I started coaching, it quickly became clear that this work had the potential to reach far beyond the individuals I was directly helping. Every client who achieved a breakthrough, who transformed their relationship with food and health, became a beacon of possibility for others in their circle. The changes were often so profound that they couldn't help but share their journey, inspiring friends, family, and colleagues to consider making changes in their own lives.

I realised that to make a real, lasting impact, I needed to think bigger. My vision expanded beyond just coaching individual clients—I wanted to create a movement. A movement where people were empowered to take control of their health through food and lifestyle choices, where they were equipped with the knowledge and tools to break free from the cycle of dieting and poor health that so many find themselves trapped in.

I began to reach out to women leaders who were making a difference in various sectors—education, business, healthcare, and community work. These women, many of whom were facing their own struggles with health, were in positions of influence where their personal transformations could inspire others on a much larger scale. By working with them, I saw the potential to amplify the impact of my work exponentially.

One of the most exciting developments in my journey has been the opportunity to collaborate with other change-makers—those who are equally passionate about health, well-being, and empowerment. Together, we've started to build platforms where we can share our insights, offer support, and inspire action. Whether it's through speaking engagements, online summits, or collaborative projects, the goal is always the same: to spread the message that better health is within reach for everyone, and it starts with conscious, intentional choices.

In addition to my work with WILDFIT®, I'm now on the verge of becoming a certified Diabetes Reversal Facilitator. This certification will allow me to help even more people, particularly those dealing with the challenges of type 2 diabetes—a condition that affects millions worldwide and dramatically reduces their quality of life. The fact that type 2 diabetes can be reversed through lifestyle changes is incredibly empowering, and I'm passionate about spreading this message as widely as possible.

Looking ahead, I see a future where this movement continues to grow, reaching more people and creating lasting change. I'm open to new ideas and collaborations and eager to work with others who share this vision. I want to continue raising awareness, spreading positivity, and leading by example. The journey is far from over—in many ways, it feels like it's just beginning.

I'm committed to finding bigger platforms for change: speaking on stages, delivering training, and reaching out to communities that are ready for transformation. This is about more than just coaching; it's about starting a revolution in how we think about food, health, and our bodies. It's about creating a world where people are empowered to make choices that support their well-being, not just because they feel they should, but because they see the incredible possibilities that lie ahead.

Together, we can create a movement that changes lives—not just on an individual level, but on a global scale. I'm excited to see where this journey will take me and to continue making a difference in the lives of those who are ready to take control of their health and embrace a brighter, healthier future.

7. A New Paradigm for Health

As I reflect on the journey that has brought me to this point, I'm filled with a profound sense of purpose and excitement for what lies ahead. The transformation I've experienced in my own life—both physically and emotionally—has given me not just a new lease of life, but a clear mission: To help others discover the incredible transformational power of natural food to help them reclaim their own health and wellbeing.

I'm passionate about reaching people far and wide who are trapped in painful cycles of dieting, emotional eating, and self-doubt. Those who feel overwhelmed by the demands of modern life, eating for convenience and struggling with conditions like ADHD, type 2 diabetes, or chronic pain. They have been led to believe that their health is beyond their control, and that the only solution requires medication. I'm here to help them see that better health is absolutely within reach, by taking the right steps in the right order.

My vision is simple: I want to help more people take control of their health. I'm looking for new ways to share this message, whether that's through speaking, working with others, or creating online programmes to reach a wider audience.

I'm especially passionate about helping people reverse diabetes. It's crucial to spread the message that this condition can be reversed with the right food and lifestyle changes, not just managed.

This will need collaboration with leaders in education, healthcare, and business to make people understand the truth—eat well to feel great! Imagine teaching children to have a healthy relationship with food or workplaces that support healthy choices for their staff. These are the kinds of changes I want to drive.

Everyone knows that we are meant to be eating healthier, but they don't have a real connection to why that is. I think most of us are unaware that if you improve the way you eat right now, you will feel almost *instant* benefits. You can literally feel better *today*! That's it, simply put. Eat Well, Feel Great is my mantra, my brand, my calling.

It's not about perfection or deprivation. It's about making small, sustainable changes that lead to big results over time. It starts with connecting to your "Big Why"—the deeply personal reason that motivates you to make healthier choices, not because you feel you *should*, but because you have found your deep motivation to *truly want* to change. For me, it was about wanting to show my authentic identity of someone who is passionate about health and longevity, wanting to live a life free from the constant battle with my body and food relationship. For my clients, it's often about regaining their confidence, reducing pain, or reversing a chronic condition so that they can spend more precious time with their families. Whatever your "Big Why" may be, it's the key to unlocking a new way of living.

The next step is tuning in consciously to how foods make you FEEL. then it's about making one healthy swap at a time.

But this transformational method I teach is much more than just your typical "healthy eating". It's about knowing which foods humans evolved to eat, and understanding the principles around the four different food seasons.

Telling you what that looks like doesn't work. Creating a meal plan for you won't work. No behaviour change is as easy as simply telling someone what to do.

If you want the benefits without spending years figuring it out on your own, there's a simple way forward. Working with a WILDFIT® Master Coach like me will give you the insight and support to make the changes doable. It's about knowing the 'how'—the strategies that work with your body and life, making it a smoother, more enjoyable process for sustainable results. There are currently 10 WILDFIT® Master Coaches worldwide and many more junior coaches. If you think you'd like to work with me, reach out to me through the contact details on this page and we can have a chat about what's possible for you.

It takes 90 days to transform your health and your weight.

My average client releases 21 lbs. But more importantly, they overcome a wide range of typical symptoms such as joint pain, digestive disorders, fatigue and improve their body composition, sleep and food relationship. They never need to go on a diet again.

Once you have experienced this transformation for yourself, you will want to share it with others.

You can be part of the change and help me create a ripple effect where people are living by example, showing what's possible. When one person makes a change, it inspires others to do the same, creating a wider movement of health and vitality. By leading the way, each of us can make an impact—not just on our own lives, but on the people around us.

So, I invite you to join me on this journey. The impact we can create together is limitless.

Let's make it happen.

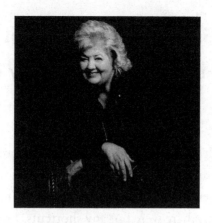

Donna J Thomas

CEO of Mountainside Gals!!!
Entreprenuer, Speaker, Podcaster & International Best Selling Author

https://www.linkedin.com/in/donnacthomas/
https://www.instagram.com/mommadonnafromthemountainside/
https://linktr.ee/MountainsideGals
https://www.mountainsidegals.com/

Donna J. Thomas, CEO of Mountainside Gals is an influencer among LuLaRoe retailers and has sustained sales among the top 10% of the company. Donna coaches and mentors her team and when she has free time, she appears as a guest on podcasts, is a podcaster, is a speaker, and is an international best seller author. She has built a sizeable active community of women who engage and uplift each other, and all share the love fashion.

Career wise, Donna has had progressive leadership advancement and built programs for women to be mentored/coached and advanced through the ranks. Her leadership as well as mothering styles are strongly inspired by her life's faith journey.

Donna challenges herself to go the extra mile in all that she does, and she aims to bless lives daily. She lives with her husband, son and nephew in the mountains of southern Frederick County, Maryland.

True Grit: A Story of Tenacity and Determination to Be Healthy & Well

By Donna J Thomas

When I was in high school, I was pretty active and stayed in good shape. However, the tide turned when I started college and found myself sitting quite a bit and then when I went to Corporate America and started climbing the ladder, there were not any shortcuts. I worked long hours and sat quite a bit working on the computer. The context of what I did was not important, but I moved into a world where I ended up getting married, having kids and learning to balance as best I could to keep the promotions and money rolling in. My husband and I decided that I needed to work, so he did not have to work three jobs to replace the income I was earning. We did not want strangers raising our kids. But not

In my late 40s, it dawned on me that when I became a grandmother, I needed to be a fun one and be able to chase them down and have outdoor play. I have always been someone to research my options, and I automatically took surgery and diet plans off the table. I did have a gym accessible to me and chose to walk on the treadmill 2 to 3 times a week – when I could, but not often enough.

In December 2012, I bought a book, highly recommended by my family doctor, and I read it in one sitting and took lots of notes. The book has more educational and factual info about health and wellness than other books I had access to as a student or a mom. It is called The China Study (the version published in 2005) by T. Colin Campbell and Thomas M. Campbell. This book contained a great oversight of nutrition across 40 years of research in many different cultures, and they give the reason why one should consider the consumption of plants, animals, etc. (Just as an aside, I would love to meet them one day!)

Also, in December 2012, I bought a Nutribullet to give to my husband as a Christmas present. To make a change like this, he needed to be open to the idea of juicing and changing our daily routine.

Based on my research, these are the choices I made to begin this journey with permanent change (if you choose to do something like this, go to your doctor and get a nutritionist involved!):

- Drink only water (use an app to figure out how much you need based on weight and BMI) and coffee (no sweetener, honey, cream or milk)

- Eat only fresh veggies, fruit and fresh meat (no antibiotics or genetically modified items). Front-load consumption with fruits and veggies and don't eat anything after 6pm ET.

- No preservatives. No condiments. Balsamic vinaigrette is my only dressing for salads.

- No processed foods. No pasta (unless it is spinach or carrot pasta, once a month). No canned, boxed or frozen items.

- Nothing white. You can have brown rice, not white. Any foods that are bleached are bad for your body. You can have eggs, but no bread.

In January 2013, I started doing a Nutribullet* for breakfast – a well-established routine in the Thomas household. * The Nutribullet has fresh veggies and fruits in it daily. I don't have recipes, but the people who created the Nutribullet blender do. After consuming between 6 and 7 in the morning, I don't get hungry again until 1pm or so.

Within one week, I had dropped about 10 pounds by trading cereal or eggs and bacon for the Nutribullet. I got bold and bought another one to take to work, and I also blended one meal for lunch. The weight loss was quick and easy – I did not exercise. I had so much weight to lose, and I did not want to deal with hip or knee issues.

When I reached the 50-pound weight loss, I worked hard to maintain that loss, so I backed off juicing and added some processed foods every other day. I found the balance I needed to maintain. Big weight losses can be detrimental, so I wanted my body to catch up. The change I have made has been very impactful on my body temperature, I run cold even in the heat of the summer and find myself wearing sweaters and leggings a bunch all year long.

I lose anywhere between 40 and 60 pounds at once and then work to maintain my loss for about 8 to 10 months before I do it again.

Over the years, I have learned about some other changes I needed to make. I drink my coffee black now, but I just recently discovered I needed to add fat back into my daily routine, so I put cream (fresh, not pasteurized) in my coffee.

No matter the choices we make, other factors play into our ability to lose. Just recently, I developed a sleeping disorder that has not been diagnosed, but I am going through a series of tests (right now, as we are getting ready for the publication of this book). The sleeping issue may be tied to anxiety*, which has progressively gotten worse. And, the doctor has shared that the last 40 pounds to lose is considered the "tough" weight that the body does not want to lose. He believes that once we can correct my sleep disorder, those last 40 pounds will permanently disappear!!! So you will have to read an update in a couple of years to see what happens. * Anxiety has never been an issue to me throughout my life, so this is also very new to me.

Along with these changes I made, I do a daily Coffee & Bible study with my husband, and I traded the Corporate America career for a work-at-home one. I am an entrepreneur, and I run a boutique (brick-and-mortar and online). All of these changes have improved my mindset and have made me more active. Staying positive helps me pursue the passions in my life with true grit.

Where was I at 647 pounds on Jan 1, 2013? Frustrated. Needed help getting off the couch or floor. Could not participate in active play.

A picture says it all. This is one of my comparison photos that show the differences. The next picture is after the last 40 pounds are gone.

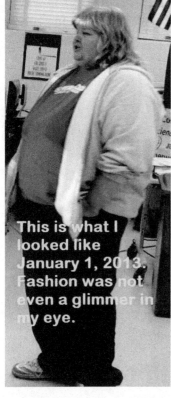

This is what I looked like January 1, 2013. Fashion was not even a glimmer in my eye.

Now, 333 pounds lighter and some to still go, I am a Trainer with LuLaRoe styling Julia with leggings (underneath) and a DeAnne skirt and a Kenny jacket.

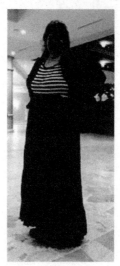

March 23, 2019

My plan is to find the answers that can help me noninvasively, meaning no surgery or special diet. The choices I have made have been wise, and I can get up from sitting down on my own, and I am able to be actively at play. I have come a long way and the journey is a permanent one for me. I was not healthy and probably did not like myself too much, either. My decision is lifelong, and I have no regrets. It has taken me a long time to reverse the tides in my life, and I like it.

Feel free to reach out to me, if you have any questions. Please understand what I did was supervised by a physician, but all changes where my own.

No dietician, no surgeon and no paid program, just true grit. The next chapter in this journey is to solve the sleeping issue and to reintroduce regular exercise on the treadmill 3 times a week, minimum. I was concerned about how heavy I was to put that additional pressure on my joints.

Thanks for learning about my journey, and I wish you well in yours.

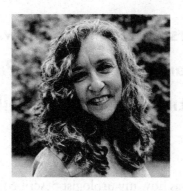

Gina Marisa

Gina Marisa Wellness
Corporate Wellness and Stress Management Expert

https://www.linkedin.com/in/gina-marisa-683534ba/
https://www.facebook.com/profile.php?id=100063743583195
https://www.ginamarisa.com/
https://unite.live/channels/gina-marisa-wellness-2/gina-marisa-wellness-603

Gina is a corporate wellness & stress management expert dedicated to helping professionals reduce stress and overwhelm into fuel for a successful career using her holistic approach. Her journey toward health began when she discovered she was in renal failure, leading to a life-saving kidney transplant 30 years ago. This experience inspired her to prioritize good health.

Gina has practiced yoga for several years and is a Level II Reiki practitioner. Through extensive research and personal health challenges, she has embraced a holistic lifestyle that integrates both body and mind. She utilizes various holistic modalities, including yin yoga, meditation, nourishment, and aromatherapy, to help her clients gain more energy and focus, improve sleep, reduce brain fog, and alleviate fatigue.

Gina is a self-proclaimed wellness enthusiast, a lifelong learner, and enjoys writing, traveling, photography, and hiking.

Resilience and Renewal:
How a Transplant Fueled a Passion for Crafting a Career in Wellness

By Gina Marisa

BIZZARE!!! That was how my urologist described my condition in my medical records that I was taking to my nephrologist (it was also underlined three times). It was not the last time I would hear that word to describe my journey to a kidney transplant, even though it did scare me to see it in print. As I write this, it seems impossible that it took place more than 30 years ago. I was having an unrelated urological issue and began seeing a urologist. While doing his workup for that condition, I had to do a 24-hour collection of my urine. When the results came back, they showed a high level of protein in my urine. This is not good.

He then sent me to have an X-ray of my kidneys. The X-ray is called an IVP, an Intravenous Pyelogram. The test is fairly easy. You are injected with a dye (the contrast) and then lay on a table while a machine takes images of your kidneys. When the doctor called me into his office to discuss the results, I wasn't thinking too much about the outcome—I mean, I was in my early 20s, healthy and not worrying about a major medical diagnosis. And even when he said he was referring me to a nephrologist, a kidney specialist, it still didn't register.

My nephrologist, Dr. Weinstein, was a very direct, no-nonsense guy—meaning his bedside manner wasn't super polished. His demeanor was completely the opposite of my urologist whom I loved (I learned years later that he opened a bagel store, which says a lot about the kind of guy he was). But since I didn't have a lot of medical "experience," it didn't occur to me to be offended. After reviewing my records he looked up and said, very nonchalantly, "Eventually, you will need a kidney transplant." I remember thinking, "What does that mean?"

He diagnosed me with dysplastic kidneys. He explained that I was born with my kidneys this way, and they worked for me for the first 23 years of my life, but they would not last forever. He said that there were a couple of things I could do to slow the inevitable transplant. My initial protocol included reducing my protein intake to four ounces per day. I wasn't really focused on a healthy diet at that point, so it seemed daunting to me to have to weigh my food. I was, however, a very good patient because I wanted to prolong the transplant as long as possible.

Apparently, my blood pressure was also high, so I had to go on medicine to keep that under control. Weighing my food wasn't particularly challenging except when I went out to eat. I remember once going to Subway at lunch. I don't know if they still do it today, but 30 years ago, they used to weigh their protein before making a sandwich, so when I ordered a tuna sandwich and requested they only put two ounces of meat on my bread, I was surprised to hear "we can't do that." Mind you, two ounces was less than the amount they normally put on a sandwich.

"So let me get this straight—I'm asking for less meat but am willing to pay the same price and you won't weigh the tuna?"

"No ma'am, we can't do that."

I was so angry that I stormed out and swore that I would never eat at another Subway. And save for one time when I was on a family trip where I wasn't driving, I have kept that promise. The low protein diet lasted for two years before my kidneys began failing to the point of needing a transplant.

The next phase of my journey was to have family members tested to see if they would be a match. Parents are automatically a half-match but siblings have a higher percentage of success. Fortunately for me, I have two younger brothers. Both were nervous about the prospect of giving up a kidney, but they both got tested. My oldest brother told me that he fainted when they took his blood, which didn't bode well for a potential major surgery, but alas, neither of them was a match.

The doctor explained that I was the perfect candidate. I was young, healthy, not overweight, and able to have a live donor—my dad. When my parents discovered one of them would be donating, they decided it would be my dad because he had short-term health insurance, so my mom was our caregiver. Then the testing began on my dad to make sure he was healthy enough to donate his kidney—which he was.

At that time, we were told I would be in the hospital for about five days and my dad would be in for about a week. The surgery is more difficult for the donor than the recipient, which always seemed weird to me. The surgery, which took place in January, went well. The most difficult aspect was having to lie on my back for the first 24 hours.

When visitors came, they had to wear a mask. This was because I was now immunocompromised and susceptible to catching everything. My recovery went well, and I left the hospital after five days, and my dad left after six. My parents were in the process of building a house at the time, so they were staying with my aunt. Since my husband was working, I stayed with my parents so my mom could be my caregiver. My aunt also helped in my recovery. The doctors wanted me to move as soon as possible, so every day my aunt would help me walk. She would hold my arm as we walked slowly down the street. At first, I could barely walk past the driveway, but in time, we walked further every day.

A few weeks after my transplant, the local newspaper reached out wanting to interview me and ask me about my experience. Transplants were not as well known as they are today, and live-related donors were less common. The main thing I remember about the interview was the picture they took. It was the first time my picture was taken (this was before cell phones) and I was shocked when I saw it. My face was round and puffy—drastically different from my pre-transplant thin and long facial structure. I hated it! I remember being in a wedding shortly thereafter and having a family photo taken. When another aunt saw the photo, she said, "Who's that girl in the picture?" I know she didn't mean any harm, but that statement was enough for me to decide right then that I would not be taking any more pictures.

My diet changed after the transplant. While I was able to eat protein again, fruits and vegetables were more work. I had to rinse everything before eating. This was to prevent me from consuming any potential bacteria. It was a pain to do, but I was very compliant because I didn't want my kidney to fail and have to go on dialysis. I was also compliant with taking my medication. There were many medications in the beginning, but slowly, as the months went by, I was able to cut back on a couple of them.

Things were moving along smoothly until August. I missed my period in July but didn't think much of it. When I missed my second period in August, I decided to take a home pregnancy test, but it was negative. A few more weeks passed and when I still didn't get my period, I went to the doctor who ordered a blood test—yep, I was pregnant. Since I was almost three months pregnant when we found out, my husband and I didn't wait long to tell my parents. We were all very excited—me, my husband, my parents, family—but the doctors were not. I remember my nephrologist telling me that I had a slim chance of becoming pregnant before the transplant, but now I was Fertile Myrtle as my mom would say!

Because of the transplant, I had to see a high-risk OB-GYN. I found a great small practice and began my pregnancy journey. I received excellent care from the two doctors who looked after me but the pregnancy was not without its challenges. I developed sciatica, which is a pain that ran from my left glute down my thigh. My insurance would not pay for the physical therapy the doctor ordered, so I was relegated to sleeping with a pillow between my legs. Genital warts were another challenge I had to endure. These were surgically removed after my baby was born. For the most part, though, my pregnancy was smooth—until week 34 when they put me on bed rest, which lasted three weeks. At week 37, I was admitted to the hospital.

My mom and husband were in the private room with me and watched the monitor while I had contractions. They told me when I was having them because I could barely feel them, which I was super excited about. I remember thinking, "Oh, this is a contraction—easy peasy!" But I wasn't progressing the way they wanted so they decided to induce me. And then, things got wild. My baby's heart rate dropped, and a flurry of activity commenced. "We have to do a C-section right now," the doctor said. A nurse gave me a small cup of liquid to drink. Another nurse gave me a shot. Aids began unhooking me from all the monitors and began wheeling me out of the room and down the hall to a surgical room. The doctor told me he was going to do a vertical incision instead of the usual horizontal incision because he didn't want to put my kidney at risk. Then the anesthesiologist put the mask over my face, and I was out.

My husband and I decided we didn't want to know the sex of our baby, so I was a little annoyed when I woke up from the anesthesia to a banner that read, "Welcome, baby girl!" I saw the banner before seeing my baby. There were also about 15 people in my room, which was really annoying. Imagine being put under, having a C-Section, and waking up groggy to a banner you didn't want to see and too many people hanging out in your tiny room. Finally, after my husband changed her first dirty diaper (from which he nearly puked when he did), I was able to hold my beautiful daughter. She had a TON of hair, which confirmed all the heartburn.

A few weeks after taking her home and loving every minute, I was lying on the couch while she was sleeping. And I remember thinking, "How am I going to do everything? I have a husband, a house, a baby, and a job. I don't know if I can do this." Years later, I realized that I probably had post-partum depression, but it really wasn't talked about back then. I somehow broke out of that on my own, and five years later, my husband and I divorced. I was fortunate to live near my parents who offered to take me and my daughter in while I saved for a place of my own. We stayed with my parents for two years, and then I bought my own house.

It was during this time that I discovered a magazine called *Body and Soul* that changed my life. It was a magazine that focused heavily on the connection between the body and the mind, as well as understanding emotions and self-healing. One column that I read religiously every month (I was hooked after reading the first issue) was by Cheryl Richardson. Cheryl's zone of genius was self-care, which wasn't something that I was practicing, at least when it came to the mindset piece. Reading her articles made me feel like I wanted to do better and be better. I began doing more self-reflection and more inner work. During my time reading the magazine, I also discovered the book, *The Secret,* which introduced me to many people who shaped the person I am today. I began reading and following the work of Joe Dispenza, Louise Hay, Wayne Dyer, Deepak Chopra, and more.

I was like a sponge with this new material and began to think differently. The mind-body connection was new to me, but it made so much sense. I grew up in an era where the mind and body were thought of as separate, meaning the mind has no effect on the body and vice versa. I eventually discovered yoga. So many people that I followed had a yoga practice that changed their life for the better. But I didn't begin there. I jumped in with both feet and decided I needed to be a yoga teacher, even though I had only taken one yoga class at my gym years prior and wasn't really a fan.

On day one of my teacher training, I began to have second thoughts about what I was doing. We had to give a short teach-back to one other person on the poses we learned that day. Wait, what?! I have to speak in front of other people? How did I miss that point? But that wasn't all I missed. The initial training to receive your certification is 200 hours, which, over a period of six months, would equate to more than one hour of yoga a day. Was I crazy?? How would I possibly fit this into my already hectic life of being a single mom? But it was too late. I already paid the fee and committed to the training. I didn't realize it at the time, but I was doing something that scared me, which turned out to be a good thing.

Over the six months, I began to notice and pay attention to my emotions. At first, I made small changes to my lifestyle. For instance, I began to practice deep breathing during my 45-minute ride to work. I prayed for other drivers on the road. When I was in public, I would send good vibes to people I passed. Gratitude was more present in my life. One day, I bought a lottery ticket at a gas station and gave it to the woman one pump over. The sheer delight on her face made me light up inside and out.

Even though my teacher training was for vinyasa, we learned about other types of yoga, such as chair yoga, restorative yoga, kundalini, and yin. While they were all useful, and I enjoyed learning about all of them, yin yoga was where I found myself. The very first time I did a yin practice we were in balasana, child's pose, and I began to cry. This felt like home, and I knew I wanted to explore this practice further.

Shortly after finishing my training, I began working with an astrologer. We discussed my desire to help others on their wellness journey using holistic methods, and she suggested taking my classes online. This idea appealed to me because I could help more people. Today, I help professionals and executives lower stress using holistic methods. Having worked in the corporate arena for over 35 years, I understand how stress and overwhelm can affect your work life, personal life, and family life.

Holistic methods work well when dealing with stress. As I mentioned, yin yoga is one of my favorite ways to regulate stress. Because you hold poses for three to five minutes, you are in a place where you can really pay attention and focus on your body. The holds are like mini-meditations, which is why I like to say that yin yoga is a dual-purpose practice.

A few months before I began my yoga teacher training, I learned about the power of aromatherapy during stressful moments. For instance, peppermint on your temples can ease head tension. And frankincense is great for reducing tension and anxious feelings. Combining aromatherapy with slow, deep inhales can instantly put your body into parasympathetic mode (rest and digest). Being in a parasympathetic state is vital for keeping stress at bay and keeping you healthy.

Chronic stress, or being in a sympathetic state (fight or flight) most of the time, impacts every part of your body, from your digestive and reproductive systems to your immune system. Eating certain foods that provide nutritional needs can calm stress hormones and keep your energy high. The benefits include more energy, a boosted immune system, which will keep illness at bay, and a calmer mind.

Through years of research and personal experience, I've come to understand that the human body is truly remarkable, with an innate power to heal itself. From maintaining a healthy kidney for 30 years to healing plantar fasciitis with specialized footwear, to alleviating tennis elbow through massage, and managing pain through breathwork, I've seen firsthand the body's capacity for self-restoration with the right mindset and approach.

My passion lies in empowering professionals and executives to reduce stress and enhance their lives through the holistic methods I've shared. These techniques often eliminate the need for pharmaceuticals or surgery, offering a natural path to well-being.

If you're ready to transform your stress into energy and focus, banish brain fog, and reclaim your vitality, I'm here to guide you. Imagine the possibilities: a well-deserved promotion, deeper connections with loved ones, more time with your kids, relief from headaches, or simply better sleep—all achievable through simple, proven strategies.

Your journey to a healthier, more balanced life could be just a conversation away. Let's work together to make your best future a reality.

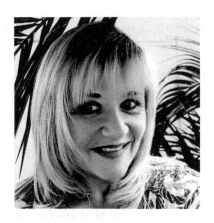

Catherine Medel

Founder of CTM Healthy Hope LLC

https://www.linkedin.com/in/catherine-medel-b07b9871/
https://www.facebook.com/catherine.medel.5
https://www.instagram.com/catarinam_author

I am a strategic licensed broker in health & life insurance with 24 years experience. I saw a need to educate as many people as possible since Healthcare & Insurance is a top issue today that's difficult to understand. I am determined to bring people HOPE (Healthy Opportunities Perfect for Everyone). I have gone through many health issues since my mid 20's & have recently published a healthy cookbook for mind body & soul. I have done research in health & wellness over many years so I could better understand my own issues & needs in order to be able to guide others on a better journey to their being healthy & wellbeing. I still learn every day & in using the best tools, with knowledge & understanding from other professionals in the same industry I feel I must share with others that are struggling to make their lives better.

The Wellness Wonderland:
Nourish and Flourish

By Catherine Medel

Wellness and healthcare are such a business now that the word "care" is usually an afterthought.

The healthcare industry is such a hot topic nowadays, whether in the political realm, a business booming career, or the newest technology breakthrough. Everywhere you turn, whether it be the media, published articles, infomercials, or even blogs you hear information on healthcare and wellness.

U.S. News & World reports that healthcare careers dominate the list of best jobs for the last several years now, even above the technology sector. It's due to the combination of high salaries, lower unemployment rates, and better work-life balance. And now since the pandemic in 2020, healthcare occupations are in such demand and expected to grow even more in the future due in part to the amount of baby boomers that are in the senior generation now. However, our healthcare system doesn't seem to be improving in many ways unless there's usually a price tag attached to it.

According to the CDC (Centers for Disease Control), statistics show that roughly 1 in 75,000 American deaths are caused or influenced by infections picked up in hospitals. Protocols governing basic sterilization procedures have been put in place since 2009, but still, healthcare bureaucrats and even physicians refuse to follow protocol. They see it as an intrusion or an unnecessary procedure. So, how is it that a single illness from a piece of food can close down a food business, yet be tolerated as an afterthought of "care" in a healthcare facility? But it's not just a facility or physician that has bad practices, it's the process that has grown over many years. Whether it's the greed of the pharmaceutical companies, unaffordable prices of health insurance, political leadership's ignorance, or tired, worn-out healthcare workers. It seems no one is willing to solve the real issues and problems because the reforms of legislation, paperwork, and runaway costs of this industry are difficult to deal with.

I work in the healthcare industry and, for years, have seen things done wrong in many aspects. It seemed most of the time I tried to speak up, I received pushback and was told to mind my place. Incentives given by government plans, commercial plans, or business-governed provider offices are designed basically as dollar-driven incentives so that it "seems to be about caring for the patient's well-being," but in essence, it's to bring in more money for the company. I hear many consumers speak of how messed up our healthcare system is, most don't even understand the causes of the problem. One thing I do understand is that the system would rather emphasize treatment over prevention, and unfortunately, many consumers in our country allow it. They get frustrated over costs and lack of care from their doctor or facility and staff but would rather not deal with trying to do something healthy to reverse or avoid the health issue to begin with. Do you realize that it's easier and cheaper for a family of 3 or more to eat at a fast food restaurant (i.e., McDonald's) or buy food at the grocery store that's less healthy than to buy the healthier organic type of food to help prevent the disease/illness in the first place?

When will we take back control of our own lives and think about the "care" of our health??

Promoting the nation's health and well-being is a shared responsibility on all levels. Health is defined as "a state of complete physical, mental, and social well-being and not merely the absence of disease or illness."

People often use the terms health and wellness interchangeably. Although you cannot have one without the other, it's two different concepts that have different meanings. The primary difference between health and wellness is that health is the goal, and wellness is the process of achieving it. You can't have health without achieving wellness first because overall health is directly influenced by wellness.

There are 6 areas of wellness that affect our health.

1. Physical: Exercise and good nutrition are essential parts of health in order to prevent illness and disease.

2. Intellectual: Mental exercise to challenge our minds helps create a better life and avoid mental health problems.

3. Emotional: A person with emotional wellness can deal with stressful situations and learn to have empathy and self-esteem.

4. Environmental: Awareness of nature and keeping our environment free of hazards promotes wellness.

5. Social: Support networks, along with contributing to the community, will bring health and happiness to people.

6. Spiritual: Developing compassion and caring brings purpose to spiritual wellness, it doesn't imply religion or faith... It's spiritual healing.

By the time I was in my 20s, I was beginning to have issues with digestion and overall stomach problems. I went through many diagnoses and dealt with lots of digestive illnesses. I dealt with different illnesses for decades, and they caused me physical, mental, and emotional pain, anxiety, depression, and overall very extreme problems. I started researching in my 30s to see what was causing all these problems and looking for a "cure" because I was sick and tired of being sick and tired. I started researching gut health, herbs, and natural items that could get to the root of the problems with my stomach and digestive system. Wow, I was overwhelmed with all the information out there and didn't really know what to believe or trust that would truly be the answer. I say that now because for 15 or more years (2005–2022), I was told by several doctors that I had Crohn's disease after I had dealt with IBS and Ulcerative Colitis years before that. I took the drugs, steroids, and blood transfusions they had me on for almost 5 years!! What an even bigger mess my life became because of these "fixes." I decided to change my life, lifestyle, and attitude and again started researching natural things to get my life back. So, my new journey began, and I stopped eating sugar, fast food, processed foods, and other things that I knew were not necessarily good for me or triggered my digestive issues. I started eating Mediterranean style, drinking water, and quitting the Cokes. I started noticing a difference, so I added exercise by taking fast, hard walks about 3 times, 15 miles, a week. This started reversing my issues, and within 10–11 months, I lost the 110 lbs I had put on from the steroids and depression. My blood work started going in a positive direction, and I had reversed the issues and started an exercise routine as well as eating clean and healthy.

I continued this success for about 11 years, and in 2022, it felt like "déjà vu" all over again. I started getting sick, and my physical as well as mental and emotional well-being was plummeting again. I had doctor appointments and was told that my bloodwork was dropping, and I was in the stroke and heart attack area. I went on like this for months as the doctors did procedures, and I was put in the hospital in April 2022 by the specialist. It saved my life for that moment because I almost died that night in the ER. That specialist and my surgeon had finally, after months, determined I never had Crohn's, there was no indication of it, but instead, I had a hiatal hernia all those years, and it had started growing larger over the last few years. By August 2022, I had to go into surgery because it had developed "tentacles" that wrapped around my esophagus and pulled my stomach out of my abdomen, and my stomach was on my left lung, thus collapsing it. I had the surgery, 3 days in the hospital, and 12 months of recovery. Fast forward to today, my physical, mental, emotional, and spiritual health is great. I'm so grateful for the support of family and friends, along with blessings from God to be able to be here writing, and hopefully, this will inspire whoever is reading it to become healthy. It's SO worth it!!

As time goes on, we're learning how diet plays a fundamental role in social, emotional, and mental health, specifically for health and well-being. Although there's still much to uncover about the underlying relationship between diet and mental health, there is compelling evidence that suggests the two are, in fact, very closely related. Diet and nutrition affect the way people feel mentally, and in supporting treatments of diet and lifestyle changes, these conditions can be reversed—I'm proof of that. It makes perfect sense that the foods we eat have just as much effect on our brains as it does on our bodies. One reason food choices affect the brain so strongly is that our "gut" is actually very closely connected to the brain. In fact, it's recently been referred to as "the second brain." You see, it's full of trillions of living microbes that have many functions in our body. They're called neurotransmitters, and they send chemical messages to the brain to regulate sleep, pain, appetite, mood, and emotion. Makes sense, doesn't it??

For several years, many studies have linked diet and gut health with the risk of depression. One study found a diet rich in fruits, vegetables, whole grains, and legumes, along with less eating of processed and red meats, lowers the odds of depression symptoms. So, for depression issues, eat a Mediterranean Diet. This is what I've done for over 15 years now. Also, for stress and anxiety, limit alcohol, caffeine, and sugary foods. Sugar in any form is one of the most harmful foods we can put in our bodies, so try to find other ways to satisfy your sweet cravings. Research has also shown that there's a link between anxiety and a high intake of saturated fat, low intake of fruit, and poor diet quality overall. Ultra-processed foods are those that have undergone industrial processing techniques and seem to be one of the worst foods that may harm your mental health. They tend to be higher in calories, salt, added sugar, and unsaturated fats. Eating ultra-processed foods regularly has been linked with a higher incidence of symptoms associated with anxiety, depression, and stress.

One of the most common nutrients missing from people's diets is fiber. When a diet is lacking in fiber, fat loss and healthy living goals can come to a halt. There are two types of fiber: soluble, which dissolves in water, and insoluble, which promotes intestinal movement. Both are necessary for overall health, but more importantly to shuttle waste out of the body.

An average intake of fiber from both sources for men should be around 30–40 grams daily, and for women, 25–35 grams. When these needs are not met, a host of problems arise, from poor digestion to fat storage to constipation. None of this supports a healthy lean body.

By adding fibrous foods to your diet, you will be healthier, eliminate toxins more quickly, stabilize blood sugar and cholesterol levels, and stay fuller for longer periods of time. One of the quickest ways to aid fat loss is to add vegetables to every meal and snack. From smoothies with spinach to omelets with peppers, onions, and mushrooms, the morning is a great way to add in these healthy carbohydrates. Never forget the importance of fiber for lifelong health and wellness. Besides long-term health, fiber could literally be the missing link in your fat loss plan.

Here are some examples of healthy food swaps:

- Whole foods instead of packaged and processed foods
- Whole grains instead of refined grains
- Whole fruits instead of dried fruits and juices
- Seafood or lean poultry instead of red and processed meats
- Fermented dairy instead of sweetened dairy
- Fruit-infused waters instead of sodas or energy drinks
- Kombucha or herbal tea instead of alcohol
- Herbs and spices instead of sugar and salt

There's still much to learn, but it's become clear that gut health and bacteria in the gut play a significant role in mental and physical health. I want to urge everyone who reads this book to do their own research and seek help if you're suffering from any type of physical or mental health issues.

Just one more thing I would like to say... Please try this today, I DARE YOU!

Challenge yourself to think of one food swap you can make to incorporate more fruits, vegetables, and whole grains into your diet. Your physical and mental health and well-being will thank you for it.

Sometimes, things are put into motion that you have no control over, but it doesn't mean life is over. Pick yourself up and realize you can do it no matter what it is. Wellness is a Wonderland, so Nourish and Flourish!!

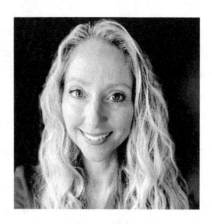

Megan Waite

Founder of Megan Waite Coaching

https://www.linkedin.com/in/meganwaite/
https://www.facebook.com/MeganWaiteCoaching/
https://www.instagram.com/meganwaitecoaching/
www.meganwaitecoaching.com

After 25+ years serving in the Health and Wellness Industry, helping people just like you and I achieve their health and wellness goals, I am proud to announce the #1 major common denominator amongst all those who achieve and sustain their goals and those who do not. I am a physical therapist and National Board Certified Health & Wellness Coach. I am also secretly a leader in a real estate investing niche. I lead from the front no matter how vulnerable that feels. I've worked with Moms, Dads, kids, families, employees, insurance companies, individuals, groups, in-person, virtual, after both minor and major life health and/or wellness events. Come discover the #1 game changer in finally sustaining your goals. My chapter is titled Your Self Care Movement. To your success! Best, Coach Meg.

Your Personal Self-Care Movement

By Megan Waite

Have you ever had moments when you feel like the world is almost your oyster? If only this one last piece would come together for you. Almost bliss, then the next moment, it feels like your world is completely falling apart? Aghhhh. The worst. Just when you think you can celebrate a milestone, something goes wrong. Yup, I get that. I've been there more times than I can count. I'm a Mom of 4 kiddos, if that tells you anything. They range from kindergarten all the way up to just starting college. I'm no spring chicken. I'm nearing my big 50th birthday! I've worked for both myself and for corporate America HealthCare companies serving in direct client care. I've had more highs and lows than I have time to share.

Let's Get Personal

Hey there! My name is Megan. People call me Meg in my professional life, but I'll answer to both. I'm a bit in awe as I report to you, that I've spent a quarter of a century in the Health and Wellness arena, helping others achieve their goals. I've supported woman just like you while we focused on everything from sick care to wellness care, from personal care goals to professional growth goals. The development of virtual meetings has allowed me to work with thousands of individuals and hundreds of companies during this time. I've taught at Universities, partnered with insurance companies, led workshops and seminars, coached programs with both individuals and groups, taught in lower-grade schools, coached aspiring students, created several proprietary programs, and always tracked my clients' results. I became a Physical Therapist in 1999 and started health and wellness coaching in 2011. I sat with the first cohort and passed the National Board Exam for Health and Wellness Coaches in 2014, and remain board-certified today.

Take Ownership Today

I've taken my 25 years' worth of work and am thrilled to have this opportunity to offer you my most impactful game changers to take ownership of your health and wellness. I can't wait to hand you my most effective and sustainable quick actions that you can implement immediately, right now, no matter where you are starting your journey into improved health and wellness. Holding a large portfolio of options in your bag of health and wellness possibilities is so helpful when one option isn't working as you'd expect. Now, for the hard truth. There is not one singular solution that works for the masses. We truly are all individuals with unique idiosyncrasies. Our bodies are supposed to respond in a particular way according to science and all the research. But, if you've ever heard a pharmaceutical list of disclaimers on television commercials, you know, there are huge variables in outcomes even with the best of the best solutions for different body types.

Why is this? Why does one solution that works so well for your friend, not work for you? That's so frustrating. When you need it to work more than anything, and you can't seem to figure out how to make it work for you. Now keep in mind, it's not you. It's likely the solution that you have chosen or perhaps defaulted to choose. Or sometimes we keep doing the same thing expecting different results. This is the definition of insanity, and I've been there myself at times, haven't you?

There is NO Perfection In It

I'm not sure if you are aware, but being healthy and happy is not a degree you earn once, and then you are complete. Your health and wellbeing are truly a daily actionable effort. Many call it a "daily practice". Practice is just a series of actions that build on each other over time. This word "practice" gives you the freedom to do as you choose and practice what you want. We all practice both the good, the bad, and the ugly each and every day. Practice means there is no perfection in it, ever. Perfection does not exist and is truly the enemy of execution. So take the idea of perfect action and toss it to the sideline. Seriously. Go ahead and write in the margins, "There is NO perfection in daily health & wellness action".

Where Are You Now

Super. Now that we have the idea of perfection tossed out, we can re-focus on some tangible actions. It's more about what you do well, most of the time. What do you practice the majority of the time? Do you practice purposeful action? If you do or if you do not, this does not matter. But let's start from where you are now. Take a moment to write down what your current routines are regarding your overall health and wellness. Let's get it out of your head and onto paper or even type it into your notes on your phone so you can take a good look at what you are currently doing. You are doing something with your time, whether your time spent is propelling you in the direction you want or not is a different conversation for later in this chapter. First, go ahead and start writing or typing. This may be a short list or a quick thought. You may write a whole paragraph. Remember, there is no perfection in it, but jot down what you're currently up to that you believe supports your health and wellness lifestyle, wishes, goals, and/or vision.

Knowing what you are currently up to that supports your health and wellness goals is such a helpful place to start in order to map out where you want to go and how you want to get there. For the sake of time, let's stay a bit general here. Where do you want to go with your health and wellness? We can do a deep dive on this, but right now, I'm going to take a risky wild guess and assume you basically want to feel better, feel happier, and enjoy each day as it comes. Am I right? To oversimplify, all of my thousands of clients over the years shared that they were working hard to meet their goals in hopes that they would feel better and be happier after the goal was accomplished. I would guess this is the same generalization for you too. Yes?

In the interest of time, let's say this is true for you too. You want to feel better and be happier.

So how do you do that? How do you get there?

Your #1 Actionable Item

How do you go from where you are now with your current state of health and wellness and achieve your general goal of feeling better and living a happier life? I want to share this answer with you. It's the jump start you have been seeking and it's probably been right in front of you the entire time. Every client who has added this actionable plan into their life has seen positive results towards feeling better. This is my most effective top hack that you can start using as quickly as today. Here is the #1 actionable item that will determine your successful outcome on your health and wellness journey. Write this down, "Self-Care IS my personal Health and Wellness care". Soak that in. I am going to repeat it. Self-care is my personal health and wellness care.

Seems simple, or is it? First, look back at this statement as your daily reminder. Write it on a sticky note and stick it on your fridge, your computer, or even your bathroom mirror. Make it your screen saver on your phone or add it to your calendar and place it on daily repeat. You can never have enough reminders until you make this statement automatic and your own.

Feeling Guilty?

Now comes a closer look. It's question time again. Do you take good care of yourself? I mean, do you give yourself time, care, and nurturing, preferably first thing in the morning, to fuel you into your day ahead? Here's something to explore. How do you show up for yourself and fill your bucket throughout the day so that you can be the best version of yourself for your job, your family, your friends, and your community?

Does this topic make you uncomfortable? Newsflash! Okay, this isn't really a newsflash, but hear this. It IS your individual right as a human to choose your personal self-care before anyone else's without guilt. Wowza. "Without guilt". Pause at the end of the statement. I find this to be quite difficult for women. To practice self-care without guilt. I know it certainly stirs an uncomfortable button for me. Here comes my vulnerable truth. I already know this information and totally failed to put my health and wellness first recently with my family. My health and wellness went down the tubes because of my own personal self-neglect.

A HUGE Price to Pay

I burned out this year when the real S*** hit the fan in my life. It is called having TEENAGERS. I had heard stories of this species of human. I felt like I had prepared for this era and was well-equipped. I actually felt like I was handling all the new adulting progressions with lots of grace and fluidity while maintaining boundaries and recognizing the teachable moments. I had thought that I had prepared myself as a parent leading up to this phase of life. I was good at being a Mom of pre-schoolers, elementary, and even middle school kiddos. I thought I was on track with raising my high schoolers. But somewhere in between running my growing business, driving kids to activities, giving time in the community, supporting my aging parents and my sister who's about to have her second child, forget trying to clean the house or love on my life partner, I forgot to keep putting myself first and lost grasp of my personal wellbeing.

You can only give as much love to others as you give to yourself. Love and caring flow outward from you and if you haven't given yourself any love to pull from, it gets depleted fast. I had forgotten to give time to myself and prioritize my personal health and wellness. Yes, this truly just happened. What came next, you ask? Oh, the big bottoming-out spiral that sends you into the depths of feeling great overwhelm, despair, and out of control. I felt terrible. I gained weight, my joints hurt, I had a foggy head, my body ached, I was consuming a sugar and carb diet, I was awake for 2 hours every night around 3:00am, I had heart palpitations, anxiety, deep sadness, and total fatigue. Forgetting to place purposeful time in my day for my own self-care was truly a huge price to pay.

If you have ever forgotten to put yourself first, your self-care first repeatedly each day, then this is your #1 place to start with the most benefit. So what does functional, on-purpose self-care look like? Honestly, it looks different for everyone. For me, it changes every day based on time, energy, and sleep, but here are my ideal self-care actions each day. My own purpose fueling self-care is a quiet cup of coffee with yoga flow music, then go to my yoga mat for a 10–15 minute mediation and yoga stretch. It's a 30-minute walk outside after I get my younger kids on the bus. It's joining a women's co-working space to get out of the house and connect with like-minded women. It's taking an exercise class 3–4 times a week. It's drinking water throughout my day. It's honoring my preferred bedtime of 9:00pm. It's not skipping meals because I'm too busy and making sure to consume protein, fruit, and veggies. It's taking my vitamins. It's committing to seeing a friend once a week even if I don't have the time. It's taking the whole day for me once a month at a spa, hike, drive, retreat, anywhere.

Let's Explore Together

I invite you to explore what your selfcare looks like for you. Here are some more ideas: writing a list of 10 things you are grateful for, enjoying a glass of water then stretching or doing some yoga. It may be going for a morning walk, taking a 20-minute hot shower or bath, listening to some soul-lifting music as you get ready for your day, cooking a hearty breakfast for yourself, or taking the time to enjoy a smoothie, or sit and nourish with something you prepped the night before. It may be simply breathing, walking in a garden, listening to the birds, watching the sunrise, washing your face daily, lotioning your body, caring for your feet, or massaging your hands. You can see these are all simple, loving actions towards yourself. Make a quick list or write about your vision for your best self-care on a time budget. Include items that are quick and can be implemented daily. Add items that may take more time or funding, so they may be included monthly or quarterly. I truly encourage you to sit for the next 10 minutes dreaming about your self-care plan that will support your goal of feeling good and being happy. You can spend as much time here as you choose.

Unveil Your Truth

If you were to place a percentage around this actionable item, "Self Care IS your Health and Wellness Care", what percentage of days in the last 30 days would you say you gave yourself even a few minutes of refueling self-care? Was it 10%, 20%, 50%? Our personal health and wellness success starts with our own self-care and thrives with 100% or 30 out of 30 days, giving even just a few minutes to our own personal self-care. The more you can give 30–60 minutes a day to yourself, the more likely you will feel healthier and happier overall. Once in this space, you have the stamina and resiliency to tackle those next-level health and wellness goals for sustainable change.

You Choose

My clients say they experience a new energy, a new jump in their step. You may experience a new resiliency when it comes to dealing with issues that arise in your day. More calmness in your body, happiness in yourself, and perhaps with your family or roommates if you live with others. Clients report they have more energy and focus to take purposeful action on their next-level health and wellness goals around exercise, diet, and more. You'll also notice a direct correlation to how you feel when you miss a day. Take note! How is your day different? Clients express feeling more negativity in their day and a sense of increased self-blame or self-disgust. If you constantly practice negative self-talk, will you ever feel true love towards yourself? Very unlikely, right? I call it "choices by the moment". You can always choose to make a change. In fact, you can start right now.

"Self-Care IS your Health and Wellness Care", has been the #1 actionable game changer for myself and my clients. If you are truly committing to yourself, you'll need to adjust your routine and likely morning habits. You may also need to prep for the morning the night before, which takes some planning ahead. This may be going to bed earlier, prepping your hearty morning meal, or notifying your family of this change. Maybe you'll choose to go to the office 30 minutes later to fit in your self-care time each day or set your alarm for 30 minutes earlier than currently. I not only challenge you to place yourself first but dare you not to. How's that working out for you? Wink :)

Gift Yourself 30 Days

Gift yourself and your new self-care routine, habit(s), or practice 30 days to soak up all its benefits. Again, there's no perfection in it. You may miss a day of self-care but try to end each day with something that nourishes just your soul only. You may push your self-care out to later in the day if you wake up late (but you'll find that won't likely be your favorite day).

Health and Wellness does not need to be complicated. Truly, it can be as simple and impactful as this #1 action of implementing a daily practice of self-care. If you have ever worked with me in the past or if you are just beginning to follow me now, you'll notice that making choices that serve your ultimate goals comes from a simple process I teach all of my clients. Unfortunately, we don't have time for the deep dive here, but let's give you the bird's eye view of what comes next so that you can pull another nugget into your treasure box.

The Simple Seven

First, your body already has innate wisdom and genius inside. If you listen, it will tell you what it wants. I had started a business back in 2011 called Body Talk. Meaning, your body talks to you. It's your job to listen and decipher what it means. You have all the genius inside you. Let's uncover it.

Second, there is always an order of operation for the highest outcomes. Meaning, if you start with publishing the book, before it's written, well … no brainer there. You have nothing to publish. There is always an order in nature, and it's no different with your body. You just need to know the order of operation for your goal(s).

Third, much of your power lies within your awareness. Would you agree? If you are not aware that this action is not helpful towards our goals, how can you choose to make a change? It must begin with being present, aware, and that uncomfortable word, "feeling". Meaning, how do you feel when you do X, Y, and/or Z? Paying attention and increasing your awareness fuels your personal power.

Fourth, being outcome-focused or goal-focused helps you know where you want to go with your actions. What are you truly trying to achieve? This helps you laser in on your choices and, in turn, reveals decisions with more ease in support of your goal(s), even if it's the harder decision.

Fifth, you must know WHY you want the goal(s) you have chosen. If your reason does not line up with what you want or does not ultimately feel good, then you have a disconnect on your path. You will have great trouble achieving your goal(s) without acknowledging your deeper why and aligning your goals. This does not mean you've failed, it simply means you have some more exploring to do.

Sixth, don't forget to execute your action plan. You spend all day reading this amazing book with kick-ass ideas that would totally change your life! But if you do not execute your action(s), you will not achieve your goal(s), and you'll spiral right back down that negative staircase. Remember, action is tangible. It's not a pie-in-the-sky action. It starts with self-care, and then, we add on.

Last but not actually least, is step seven. You must reassess and review your progress towards your goals. Has your why changed? Has your awareness changed? Are you headed in the right direction? Do you need to revisit and adjust your rudder left or right? This is a pivotal step in reaching your goals. Come on, you know what to do. Your body is genius, remember?

It's Better Together

Now, you are never alone in this. These Simple Seven steps to jump-starting your health and wellness journey and finally creating actual lasting change do not need to be taken by yourself. I've created a group just for you and your friends as you take tangible actions to live your healthy happy life.

What is your health and wellness promise to yourself? Start with the new or renewed knowing that "Self-Care is your Health and Wellness Care". As mentioned, I use a specific process to help you stay on track and measure your progress along the way. I'll be offering a deep dive into this lifelong expansive tool in my book, released in 2025. In the meantime, come grab instant support, ideas, and community over on my Facebook page. Come say "Hi!". I have a free gift ready to send, so come say hello so I can get it to you. I'll be on the lookout for you, but until then, here is your first moment of recognized freedom of choice. Put down this book to grab your gift and say "hello?" Or not? As always, it's totally your choice. Here's to knowing that "Your Self-Care is your Health and Wellness care", and it begins with your first action. To your continued health and wellness success. Cheers!

Big hugs,
Meg

JOIN THE MOVEMENT!
#BAUW

Becoming An Unstoppable Woman
With She Rises Studios

She Rises Studios was founded by Hanna Olivas and Adriana Luna Carlos, the mother-daughter duo, in mid-2020 as they saw a need to help empower women worldwide. They are the podcast hosts of the *She Rises Studios Podcast* and Amazon best-selling authors and motivational speakers who travel the world. Hanna and Adriana are the movement creators of #BAUW - Becoming An Unstoppable Woman: The movement has been created to universally impact women of all ages, at whatever stage of life, to overcome insecurities, and adversities, and develop an unstoppable mindset. She Rises Studios educates, celebrates, and empowers women globally.

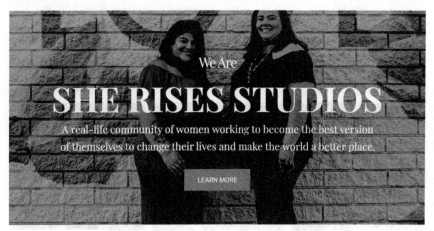

Looking to Join Us in our Next Anthology or Publish YOUR Own?

She Rises Studios Publishing offers full-service publishing, marketing, book tour, and campaign services. For more information, contact info@sherisesstudios.com

We are always looking for women who want to share their stories and expertise and feature their businesses on our podcasts, in our books, and in our magazines.

SEE WHAT WE DO

OUR PODCAST   **OUR BOOKS**   **OUR SERVICES**

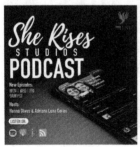
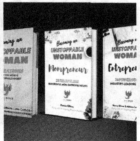
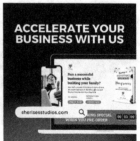

Be featured in the Becoming An Unstoppable Woman magazine, published in 13 countries and sold in all major retailers. Get the visibility you need to LEVEL UP in your business!

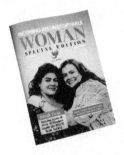 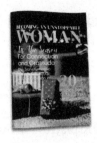 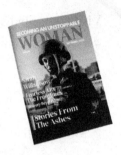

Have your own TV show streamed across major platforms like Roku TV, Amazon Fire Stick, Apple TV and more!

Learn to leverage your expertise. Build your online presence and grow your audience with FENIX TV.
https://fenixtv.sherisesstudios.com/

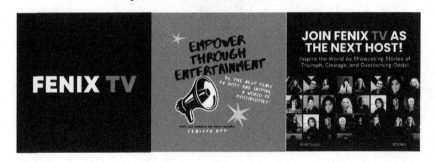

Visit www.SheRisesStudios.com to see how YOU can join the #BAUW movement and help your community to achieve the UNSTOPPABLE mindset.

Have you checked out the *She Rises Studios Podcast?*

Find us on all MAJOR platforms: Spotify, IHeartRadio, Apple Podcasts, Google Podcasts, etc.

Looking to become a sponsor or build a partnership?

Email us at info@sherisesstudios.com

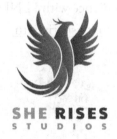

Made in the USA
Columbia, SC
28 May 2025

58514092R00102